Constant Craving A-Z

— A Simple Guide to Understanding and Healing Your Food Cravings —

DOREEN VIRTUE, Ph.D.

H
LIFE
Styles

Hay House, Inc.
Carlsbad, CA

Published and distributed in the United States by:
Hay House, Inc., P.O. Box 5100, Carlsbad, CA 92018-5100 • (800) 654-5126 • (800) 650-5115 (fax)

Edited by: Jill Kramer   *Designed by:* Wendy Lutge

Library of Congress Cataloging-in-Publication Data

Virtue, Doreen
    Constant craving A-Z : a simple guide to understanding and healing
your food cravings / [Doreen Virtue].
      p. cm.
    ISBN 1-56170-571-3 (hardcover)
    1. Compulsive eating—Popular works. 2. Food preferences—
Psychological aspects—Popular works. 3. Weight loss—Popular
works.   I. Title.
RC552.C65.V556   1999
616.85'26—dc21   98-26291
                                                CIP

ISBN 1-56170-571-3

02 01 00 99   4 3 2 1
First Printing, January 1999

Printed in Hong Kong

Contents

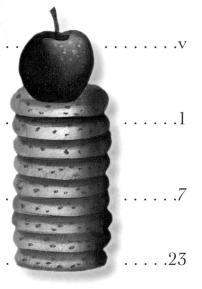

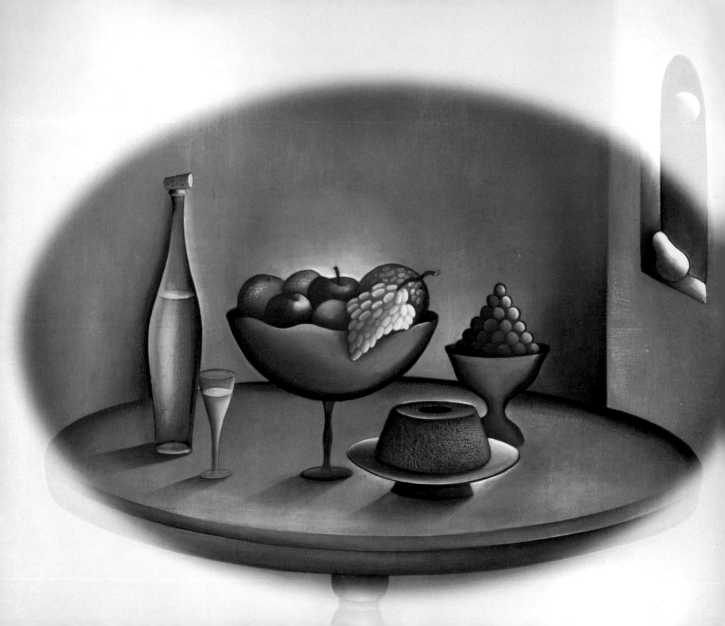

Introduction

Taking Charge of Your Food Cravings

This is a book for anyone who wants to lose weight and maintain that weight loss through the natural process of appetite reduction. *Constant Craving A–Z* brings together many years of scientific, psychological, and metaphysical research about food cravings. I wrote this book so you can interpret and reduce emotional overeating.

My education about weight and appetite stems from firsthand experience: I lost 50 pounds more than 16 years ago and learned that maintaining weight loss hinges upon maintaining peace of mind. I've also worked with hundreds of women and men across the country, helping them naturally reduce their food cravings.

I first became interested in the study of appetite because of my own struggles with cravings for ice cream and bread. As the daughter of a Christian Science practitioner mother, and a father who wrote and edited inspirational books, I knew that we are born perfect, in the image and likeness of our Creator. Physical and mental problems stem from psychological sources. False beliefs, unloving thoughts, and fear-based expectations breed illness, accidents, and disease.

Through many years of personal and clinical research, I learned the reason why I was so hungry all the time: I was afraid to trust myself. My gut was telling me to make changes in my marriage and career, and I was afraid to trust those feelings—I thought I'd fail! So I poured food on my gut to dampen its volume.

When I finally listened to my gut instead of smothering its voice with food, my life radically shifted. I transformed from a fat, unhappy housewife with no money or love in her life, into a trim-figured psychotherapist rich in friendships, love, and financial success. I learned that our gut never fails us; it is we who fail to heed its wisdom and trust its guidance.

After that, I devoted myself to studying eating disorders, overeating, and the psychological issues triggering food cravings. I discovered that each food craving corresponds to a particular personality style and emotional issue. I began sharing my food-craving interpretations with workshop audiences and clients—with remarkable results. Instead of spending hours, days, or months uncovering an emotional issue, food-craving interpretations bypass defense mechanisms and go straight to the heart of the matter. The result of all my research is now in your hands. Here is the information you need to really get honest with yourself about *why* you are craving certain foods. I've also packed in lots of suggestions and helpful advice about ways to prevent eating binges, reduce emotional eating, and regain a balanced appetite.

The journey from overeating to normal eating isn't simple, but it is necessary. To me, it's a choice between imprisonment in a "fat cell," and freedom in a light spirit and light body. I hope, like me, that you'll choose to break free from the fat cell.

— Doreen Virtue, Ph.D.

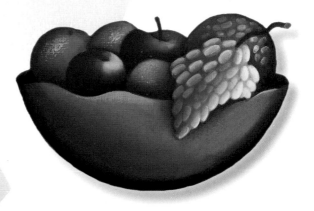

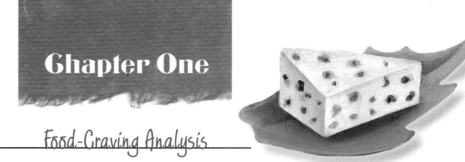

Chapter One

Food-Craving Analysis

Some people's food cravings remain constant; for example, they always crave ice cream. Other people go through "food kicks," craving peanut butter one week, blue cheese dressing the next week, and chocolate bars the following week. Neither situation is accidental nor coincidental.

If your emotional issues remain unaddressed, your food craving will remain constant. If your emotional issues change, so will your food cravings. The only parallel between both the constant and the changing food cravings is this: There is some underlying emotional issue crying out for your attention.

By "emotional issues," I don't necessarily mean deep psychological matters requiring therapy. Food cravings often stem from basic unmet needs for fun, excitement, or love—issues most would consider "normal" and within our power to self-heal.

Emotional issues connected to food cravings usually fall into one of these categories:

- Stress, tension, anxiety, fear, or impatience
- Depression or feeling blue
- Feeling tired, having low energy levels
- Unmet needs for fun, play, excitement, or recreation; too much work and not enough play
- A desire for love, affection, appreciation, romance, or sexual satisfaction
- Anger, resentment, bitterness, or frustration
- Emptiness, insecurity, or a desire for comfort

Four emotions form the core of emotional overeating: *fear, anger, tension,* and *shame* (FATS). Fear is the root emotion in the FATS feelings. Anger, tension, and shame are all extensions of fear. We feel angry because we fear losing love in the form of something or someone valuable to us; we feel tension because we are afraid of trusting or because we've walked away from our Divine path; we feel shame because we fear we are inadequate.

These "FATS feelings" are the primary triggers for emotional overeating. Overwhelming desires to eat stem from one of these four emotions.

As a psychotherapist, I feel it's important to be honest with ourselves about our emotions. We need to face the emotion and then move on. I never recommend overanalyzing one's life or viewing oneself as a victim. Yet, the source of so much needless emotional pain is the unwillingness to face an unpleasant feeling. No one enjoys admitting, "Oh, yes, I feel insecure." But the alternative—not admitting it—is so much worse!

When we deny our strong emotions, they grow even stronger. As they gain strength, they also seek outlets. Denied emotions manifest themselves in many unpleasant ways, including food cravings, physical aches or illnesses, depression, anxiety, phobias, and sleep disorders.

The bottom line is this: As unpleasant as it is to face a negative emotion, the alternative is even more unpleasant. Everyone gets angry, upset, or jealous at some time—there's no question about it. Sometimes life circumstances or our personal choices make it tough to stay centered in peace of mind. In fact, the only question about these emotions is whether we choose to deal with them now or later.

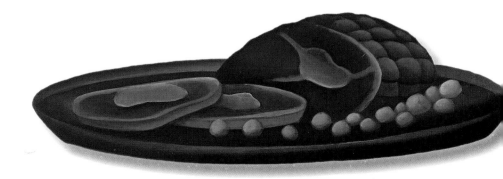

THE FOUR PRIMARY EMOTIONS
UNDERNEATH EMOTIONAL OVEREATING

FEAR   Insecurity, walking on eggshells, generalized fears, abandonment fears, existential fears, control issues, sexual fears, worry, anxiety, depression, intimacy fears.

ANGER   At another person, toward an injustice, toward self, feeling betrayed, feeling ripped off, feeling abused.

TENSION   Stress, frustration, old anger turned into bitterness, old anger turned into resentment, jealousy, impatience, overwork without an emotional release such as fun.

SHAME   Self-blame, low self-esteem, self-loathing, lack of trust in one's own competence or goodness, assuming other people won't like you, feeling less than other, feeling like you don't deserve good.

When we bottle up our strong emotions, it's akin to putting a cork on a vinegar-and-baking soda combination. The ignored emotion doesn't go away—it intensifies. The more we try to ignore a feeling, the stronger it grows. It's so much easier to face the music while the emotion is still in a "fixable" stage.

That's why I really like food-craving analysis. You start by identifying the food you crave and work backward, like a detective. Once you've identified the food you crave, say, rocky road ice cream, the underlying emotion stares you plainly in the face: "Resentment toward others and self. Feeling used or pressured, and desiring fun and comfort. Depression."

The truth of that underlying emotion, following a food-craving interpretation, hits most of us between the eyes. We instantly recognize, "Yes, that is the emotional issue I've been struggling with." This recognition may propel you to investigate further and take the healthy second step of asking yourself, "What makes me so frustrated or angry?" "What do I feel I'm missing out on?" and "Why am I taking my anger out on myself?" Usually, the answers appear right away.

Our denial system is incredibly effective in shielding us from honestly facing ourselves. Denial stems from a fear of admitting, "Yes, this bothers me." The consequences of this admission are even scarier—"Now I must take responsibility for making changes to correct the situation." Change is frightening, because we fear that our situation might worsen instead of improve.

Inertia and fears keep us from looking at underlying issues that create food cravings. Since this denial keeps us from seeing these seemingly obvious underlying issues, we often need to have them pointed out to us. It's relatively easy to see other people's issues; it's much tougher to be objective with ourselves. By learning to interpret your food cravings, you will be able to more readily discover these issues yourself.

Just honestly admitting to ourselves, "Yes, this is the emotion underneath my food craving" is such a tremendous relief! It feels so good to come clean with yourself, doesn't it? That emotional relief then reduces, or even eliminates, the urge to overeat.

Physically Based Cravings

Sometimes, we'll crave a food because our body is screaming out for nutrients, such as vitamins or protein. Our body is depleted, and cravings ensure that its needs are met. These are physically based cravings.

Yet, on close examination, even these cravings are rooted in emotions. Tension, the fourth FATS feelings, is the physical manifestation of stress in our lives. Stress leads to lifestyle choices that in turn lead to nutritional deprivation. Three of my clients discovered how stress-filled lifestyles robbed their body of energy and nutrients, which in turn triggered food cravings:

— Dianna's hectic schedule convinced her that she had "no time to exercise." Without regular physical activity, Dianna always felt sluggish and tired. Instead of solving the problem with a brisk walk or a bike ride, Dianna would eat foods to feel "peppier."

— Marcia's high-pressure job contributed to her overall feeling of tension and inability to relax. Marcia craved and ate bags of potato chips and pretzels to gnaw away her anxiety and tension. Junk foods rob our bodies of B vitamins, because empty calories require nutrients for digestion. When you use nutrients for digestion, without replacing them, you become nutrient deficient. Marcia was continually vitamin deficient and, therefore, continually hungry!

— Brenda used alcohol to calm her nerves. Excessive alcohol consumption contributes to lowered levels of the brain chemical serotonin. When serotonin is low, the usual result is carbohydrate cravings—which are exactly what Brenda struggled with. Her appetite for breads and pasta was out of control, and Brenda was very unhappy with her weight.

Yes, Dianna, Marcia, and Brenda all suffered from physically based food cravings. But the root of their nutrient deficiency was the FATS feeling, tension.

Tension also increases brain chemicals that lead to overeating. Dr. Sarah Leibowitz of Rockefeller University found that the hormone cortisol stimulates production of a brain chemical called "neuropeptide Y." This brain chemical is a chief factor in turning our carbohydrate cravings on and off. Here's the tension link: We produce more cortisol when we are tense!

Even worse, Leibowitz also reports that neuropeptide Y also makes the body hang on to the new body fat we produce (apparently this is some ancient biological throwback to the cave days). In other words, tension not only triggers carbohydrate cravings, it also makes it more difficult to lose any additional weight.

†O†

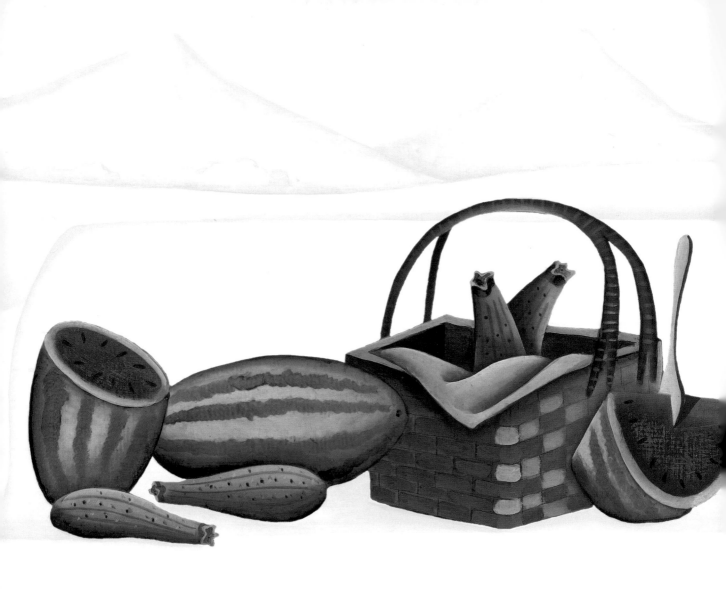

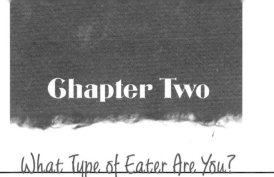

Chapter Two

What Type of Eater Are You?

Before we look further at food cravings, let's continue exploring the appetite mechanism. First, let's look at the differences between emotional and physical hunger and some of the life situations that especially trigger emotional overeating. This will help you feel more in control of your appetite and eating. You'll also be able to release any self-judgments you may be harboring about your appetite or weight once you understand the underlying reason for your eating style.

THE EIGHT TRAITS OF EMOTIONAL HUNGER

Emotional and physical hunger can feel identical, unless you've learned to identify their distinguishing characteristics. The next time you feel voraciously hungry, look for these signals that your appetite may be based on emotions rather than true physical need. This awareness may head off an emotional overeating episode.

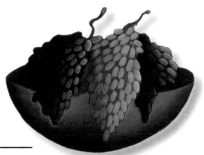

EMOTIONAL HUNGER	PHYSICAL HUNGER
1. *Is sudden.* One minute you're not thinking about food, the next minute you're starving. Your hunger goes from 0–60 within a short period of time.	*Is gradual.* Your stomach rumbles. One hour later, it growls. Physical hunger gives you steadily progressive clues that it's time to eat.

EMOTIONAL HUNGER

2. *Is for a specific food.* Your cravings are for one certain type of food, such as chocolate, pasta, or a cheeseburger. With emotional eating, you feel you need to eat that particular food. No substitute will do!

3. *Is "above the neck."* An emotionally based craving begins in the mouth and the mind. Your mouth wants to taste that pizza or chocolate doughnut. Your mind whirls with thoughts about your desired food.

4. *Is urgent.* Emotional hunger urges you to eat NOW! There is a desire to instantly ease emotional pain with food.

5. *Is paired with an upsetting emotion.* Your boss yelled at you. Your child is in trouble at school. Your spouse is in a bad mood. Emotional hunger occurs in conjunction with an upsetting situation.

PHYSICAL HUNGER

Is open to different foods. With physical hunger, you may have food preferences, but they are flexible. You are open to alternative choices.

Is based in the stomach. Physical hunger is recognizable by stomach sensations. You feel gnawing, rumbling, emptiness, and even pain in your stomach with physical hunger.

Is patient. Physical hunger would prefer that you ate soon, but doesn't command you to eat right at that instant.

Occurs out of physical need. Physical hunger occurs because it has been four or five hours since your last meal. You may experience light-headedness or low energy if overly hungry.

EMOTIONAL HUNGER

6. *Involves automatic or absent-minded eating.* Emotional eating can feel as if someone else's hand is scooping up the ice cream and putting it into your mouth ("automatic eating"). You may not notice that you've just eaten a whole bag of cookies ("absent-minded eating").

7. *Does not notice or stop eating, in response to fullness.* Emotional overeating stems from a desire to cover up painful feelings. The person stuffs herself to deaden her troubling emotions and will eat second and third helpings, even though her stomach may hurt from over-fullness.

8. *Feels guilty about eating.* The paradox of emotional overeating is that the person eats to feel better and then ends up berating herself for eating cookies, cakes, or cheeseburgers. She promises atonements to herself ("I'll exercise, diet, skip meals, etc., tomorrow.")

PHYSICAL HUNGER

Involves deliberate choices and awareness of the eating. With physical hunger, you are aware of the food on your fork, in your mouth, and in your stomach. You consciously choose whether to eat half your sandwich or the whole thing.

Stops when full. Physical hunger stems from a desire to fuel and nourish the body. As soon as that intention is fulfilled, the person stops eating.

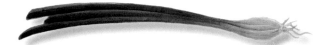

Realizes eating is necessary. When the intent behind eating is based in physical hunger, there's no guilt or shame. The person realizes that eating, like breathing oxygen, is a necessary behavior.

It takes practice and patience to consistently identify whether your hunger is emotional or physical. If you've experienced emotional hunger, you know how overwhelming that urge to eat can be. Even if you've sworn to yourself, "I'm not going to overeat," emotional hunger changes everything. Even the most committed health fanatic finds herself drawn toward the refrigerator, desperately digging for something to fulfill her cravings.

Let's break the horrible control that emotional hunger has over your appetite and eating! Let's give you back the freedom and control to say, "No, I refuse to overeat!" And the way to do that is to take these five steps the next time you feel hungry:

FIVE STEPS TO REDUCING EMOTIONAL HUNGER

The next time you feel extremely hungry, these steps may help you:

1. *Impose a 15-minute cooling-off period.* Tell yourself you cannot eat for 15 minutes. After that time, if you still feel like eating, you'll be free to do so. But during that 15 minutes, you'll be completing the other three steps, and your appetite will likely be reduced to the point where you won't want to overeat.

2. *Get away from food.* Leave the house if you must, but definitely stay away from the kitchen during the next 15 minutes. Emotional overeating often leads to "automatic" and "absent-minded" eating, where you don't realize how much food you're eating. An eating binge may be avoided simply by getting away from food. Other times, you may have to destroy the food in the garbage disposal to avoid emotional eating.

3. *If you are having "mouth hunger," brush your teeth and drink a large glass of water (but still stay away from the kitchen for 15 minutes!).* By cleansing your mouth, you can get rid of the taste of chocolate, cheeseburgers, cookies, or whatever else you're craving and help reduce your emotional appetite. The water will also help if you are confusing thirst with hunger (which occurs with surprising frequency).

4. *Ask yourself, "Am I feeling fear, or its manifestations of anger, tension, or shame?"* You don't need to go into a deep introspection over this question. Usually, the answer pops in your mind instantly, like one of those "magic 8 balls" with answers floating in the window. You'll ask the question and you'll hear the reply in your mind pretty quickly: "Yes, you're afraid about your finances," "Yes, you feel insulted by your mother's words," or "Yes, you're jealous of the way he looked at that other woman."

   Just the act of honestly admitting one's feelings is usually enough to relieve the urgency of emotional hunger. Emotional hunger is an imperative desire to cover up awareness of a painful truth, thought, or feeling. It's the equivalent of sticking your fingers in your ears when you don't want to hear something! But if you've already admitted your true feelings to yourself, you won't feel the need to run for cover in the refrigerator.

5. *Replace the FATS feelings with self-love.* We heal fear by pouring love on it. When you fill yourself with love, there is no room for negative emotions to exist. Remember the times in your own life when you were blissfully enjoying the feelings of romantic love? Remember how, during those moments, you had no desire to overeat?

   • *Look for a butterfly in your stomach.* Concentrate on your gut feelings and search for any sign of a pleasant, light feeling. Notice this feeling and ask it to expand within you, until all you feel is love, peace, and a sense of playful anticipation. Once you try this step, you'll know exactly what I mean.

- *Stay in love with this moment.* Here is an affirmation that will fill you with peace of mind if you declare it over and over:

"I Forgive, Accept, and Trust my Self."

This affirmation forms a replacement acronym for FATS, with something that is healthy and healing for you and your appetite.

The five steps above are simple, yet powerful, and you will appreciate the immediacy with which they heal constant cravings. What a wonderful alternative to fear, or its manifestations of anger, tension, and shame!

SELF-QUIZ: DETERMINE YOUR EATING STYLE

Here's a quiz to determine your eating style. When answering each question, try not to judge yourself or in any way color your answers to fit what your ideal eating style would look like.

You'll gain the most from this quiz by quickly answering each question with the first answer that pops into your mind.

WHAT'S YOUR EATING STYLE?

True or False:

1. I tend to overeat one of two certain types of food.
2. Once I have one bite of a food such as certain desserts, dairy products, baked goods, or salty junk foods, my eating and appetite go out of control.
3. I sometimes feel worried—often without reason—that I won't get enough to eat.
4. I crave certain flavors or types of foods, and sometimes the only way to make the cravings go away is to eat whatever I'm craving.
5. I have gone to extreme lengths (e.g., driven several miles out of my way, spent excessive money, etc.) to get the food I'm craving.
6. I only overeat when I'm feeling a strong emotion, such as anger or depression.
7. Right after work, I head straight for food.
8. I tend to eat whenever I'm bored.
9. Sometimes, out of the blue, I'll be incredibly hungry.
10. I feel uncomfortable openly displaying or talking about my feelings.
11. I wish I was a more confident person.
12. Just when I lose enough weight to elicit compliments or admiring glances, I start to put weight back on again.
13. I mostly want to lose weight to please my spouse, parent, lover, or some other person.
14. I'm almost to the point where I've given up hope that I'll ever lose my excess weight; maybe I'm meant to be overweight.
15. My weight makes me feel bad about myself, and when I gain weight, I feel like a failure.
16. I never seem to have enough time to eat right or exercise.

17. I'm so busy that some days I wonder if I'll drop from exhaustion.
18. I seem to be working harder these days and getting less accomplished.
19. The only way I can unwind most of the time is when I'm eating.
20. Food is a great pick-me-up when I'm feeling drained but need to keep going.
21. My weight changes during the seasons; I'm one weight in the summer and a different weight in the winter.
22. Eating is one of the few pleasures left in my life.
23. Sometimes when I'm lonely, I'll nibble on whatever's handy.
24. When I diet, I eventually stop caring whether I lose weight or not. That's when I return to overeating.
25. I often go back for second or third helpings of "diet," low-fat, or low-calorie foods.

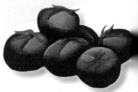

SCORING:

Add the "true" answers you gave for the following questions, and read the interpretations corresponding to your answers:

Note: There are no right or wrong answers to this quiz. It is designed to help you better understand your eating style, which is an important step in making desired behavior changes. Many people find they exhibit more than one emotional eating style—some people exhibit all five. After scoring your quiz, read the information related to every emotional eating style relevant to you.

- If you answered True to 3 or more of questions 1 through 5, you are a "Binge Eater."
- If you answered True to 3 or more of questions 6 through 10, you are a "Mood Eater."
- If you answered True to 3 or more of questions 11 through 15, you are a "Self-Esteem Eater."
- If you answered True to 3 or more of questions 16 through 20, you are a "Stress Eater."
- If you answered True to 3 or more of questions 21 through 25, you are a "Snowball Effect Eater."

FIVE CORE EMOTIONAL EATING STYLES

Did you find yourself falling into more than one eating style? Many people do. After all, we're multi-dimensional creatures who don't fit into a single pigeonhole. We are complex blends of our past experiences, heredity, present situations, emotions, thoughts, beliefs, and behaviors. We evolve and change, usually driven by desires to improve ourselves, and sometimes thwarted by life's roadblocks. All these factors influence our eating styles, and what holds true for you today may be entirely different one year from now.

1. *The Binge Eater* — This is a very black-and-white eating style — you either are a Binge Eater or you're not. Those who are Binge Eaters will instantly recognize this description.

    Certain foods trigger overeating in Binge Eaters. Those foods are often referred to as "binge foods," which are commonly made from refined white flour or sugar — foods such as sweets, pastas, and breads. Different theories have tried to explain the binge-food phenomenon. Some experts believe that Binge Eaters become anxious as a result of blood-sugar fluctuations triggered by eating high-glucose foods. This anxiety leads to a cycle of binge-eating to relieve the anxiety.

    Many Binge Eaters find that the only way to keep their appetites under control is by avoiding their binge food altogether. This is also a useful therapeutic approach, because often the binge food keeps a lid on the person's underlying emotional issues. When the binge food is removed, the emotions are free to come forward for resolution. Binge Eaters benefit from interpreting their cravings for the binge food, using the methods in this book.

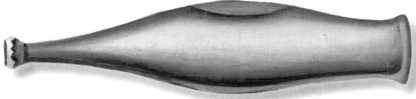

2. *The Mood Eater* — This is a person who overeats in response to strong emotions. Often, the Mood Eater is an exquisitely sensitive individual who feels a great deal of compassion for other people. She is sensitive to other people's feelings and intuitively knows when something is troubling another. Often, she is employed in a helping profession, such as teaching, counseling, or medicine.

   The Mood Eater is so filled with the emotions that she's absorbed from other people that her own emotions are ignored. She also feels overwhelmed by adding her own strong emotions onto her already full plate of other people's emotions. So she eats in order to manage her emotional capacity.

   Since the Mood Eater is a highly capable caretaker, she sometimes neglects taking care of *herself*. Sometimes she becomes upset that she is doing all the work and no one is attending to her needs. At those times, the Mood Eater feels unappreciated and resentful. She takes her frustration out the best way she knows: by eating.

   Since the Mood Eater is externally oriented — focusing more on other people than on herself — she can tune into her own feelings and become more inner-directed by interpreting her food cravings as they arise.

3. *The Self-Esteem Eater* — This is someone who uses food as a friend, a companion, and for entertainment. The Self-Esteem Eater has difficulties in interpersonal relationships. Often, she relates better to food, books, animals, and movies than she does to other people. She feels misunderstood and has been hurt by people who rejected or abandoned her. Many Self-Esteem Eaters are survivors of emotional, physical, or sexual abuse, and they learned in early childhood to distrust others.

   Much of the Self-Esteem Eater's struggle with food and weight stems from three issues:

   - *She can't bear the thought of losing her closest friend, food.* The thought of not overeating ice cream, cookies, or cheeseburgers makes her feel cold and vulnerable. If she doesn't have food for comfort, companionship, and solace, who or what can she turn to?

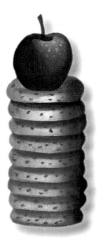

- *She has little confidence in her abilities to lead a healthful lifestyle.* The Self-Esteem Eater is usually well read and informed about the importance of healthful eating and exercise. Her library may be stocked with health books. Yet she doesn't believe she has the stamina or patience to consistently exercise. So she doesn't even try.

- *She beats herself up with eating binges.* The Self-Esteem Eater struggles with the fourth FATS feeling, shame. She questions her self-worth and wonders deep down if something is wrong with her. During these times, she punishes herself by eating to the point where her stomach hurts. The Self-Esteem Eater doesn't believe she deserves the benefits of having a healthy body.

Self-Esteem Eaters benefit more from appropriate psychotherapy than from any other style of eating. This is not to imply that something is wrong with Self-Esteem Eaters; rather, they just have the most to gain from it.

Therapy will likely be their first experience with being emotionally vulnerable to another human being. They'll be experiencing an honest and emotionally intimate relationship with a skilled therapist. When the Self-Esteem Eater finds that the therapist doesn't reject her for being herself, she will be able to connect with other people in her life. She can then develop friendships with people and stop relying on food for companionship and comfort.

The Self-Esteem Eater also benefits from food-craving interpretation as a way of becoming more honest with herself. When she faces the truth behind the meaning of her food cravings, it's a first step toward easing the loneliness that haunts her. Self-honesty always increases one's self-esteem, and food-craving interpretation is a good way to honestly confront parts of ourselves we may be afraid of facing.

4. *The Stress Eater*—This person overeats in response to the third FATS feeling, tension. I've found that two life areas trigger Stress Eating: unhappiness with one's work life and dissatisfaction with one's love life. Both life areas are difficult to change and usually take time and effort to correct. Because we can't just snap our fingers and "fix" the love or work areas, we overeat to ease the tension.

Stress Eaters display a wide range of food cravings, all intuitively chosen to ease their tension and frustration. They crave alcohol to manage their ever-taut nerves; coffee and cola to pump up their enthusiasm and energy; chocolate to ease their love-life disappointments; breads and dairy products to calm themselves down; and crunchy snack foods to ease their anger.

Food-craving interpretation is one way of accessing the underlying sources of frustration, so they may be dealt with head-on. I also encourage Stress Eaters to add four elements to their lives, which help with tension much more effectively than foods or beverages:

- *Exercise.* Please don't assume that I'm asking you to add one more responsibility to your already full plate of things to do. I realize that it's a hassle to exercise. Still, exercise is one of the easiest ways to feel better, reduce stress, get more energy, ease anger, and reduce the appetite. The best motivational tool I've ever found with exercise is to develop a firm mind-set that "exercise is a non-optional activity." Put exercise into the same category as your daily shower, and see it as something that you simply need to do. No ifs, ands, or buts!

- *Fun and recreation.* The number-one source of resentment is the feeling that everybody else gets to relax and have fun, while we're left with all the chores and work. It's a powerful residual emotion left over from childhood. Women are especially vulnerable to the notion that fun is a waste of time or a sign of weakness. Yet, fun—like exercise—is a necessity, not a luxury.

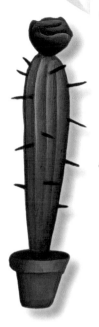

- *Time outdoors.* Stress Eaters usually lead whirlwind lifestyles. They're running at a dead heat from the moment they wake up until the time they go to bed at night. This harried pace leaves little time for noticing the simple and beautiful things in everyday life.

  If you really want to ease your tension, take a walk during your lunch hour or eat lunch outside (near grass or trees). Being outside, near nature, is instantly stress-reducing. It calms our nerves, soothes our soul, and definitely slows us down. I suppose that's where the expression, "Stop and smell the roses" came from.

- *Spirituality.* When your heart feels full of love and gratitude, very few things can get on your nerves. People who are spiritual are less vulnerable to Earthly stressors because they believe everything will turn out for the best. Instead of sweating the small details of every day life, they "let go" and trust. This doesn't mean they blindly accept the dictates of others. Spiritually guided persons are among some of the world's most successful individuals.

  All four stress-reducing elements—exercise, having fun, time outdoors, and spirituality— can be combined. Any kind of fun activity outdoors, blended with meditation or prayer, will create an incredible boost of positive feelings and energy. And when you feel great, you won't need to crave foods.

5. *The Snowball Effect Eater*—Think of a snowball rolling down a mountain, gaining speed and size, and you'll have an idea of the Snowball Effect Eater's style. This person's motivation to stick with a healthful eating and exercise program vacillates tremendously.

   Snowball Effect Eaters have inconsistent motivation levels. This is usually because their weight-loss efforts are externally motivated. They declare themselves on a diet in response to some outer stimulus, like a photograph, a spouse's comment, or too-tight jeans. These external sources of motivation just can't provide the steady stream of inspiration necessary for permanent changes in eating behavior. Internal motivation is necessary, with a focus on:

- How much energy we have when we eat healthful foods.
- How great it feels to have toned muscles.
- How exercise eases our tension or worries.
- How treating our bodies with respect leads to higher self-regard.
- How the only opinion that matters, with respect to our weight, is our own.

The Snowball Effect Eater benefits from food-craving interpretation because it keeps her anchored on internal motivations for eating. Instead of viewing her food cravings as a signal of "What's the use? I'm hungry, so I'll just abandon this stupid diet," she can understand the underlying emotional significance of her appetite.

All five styles of emotional eating can use food-craving interpretation as a means of reducing or eliminating their intrusive desires to overeat. The more you understand yourself, the more you're able to work *with*—instead of *against*—yourself. There's no need to fight yourself—that's an unloving thing to do that will only create depression and resistance within you. Instead, we're moving toward gently understanding and accepting yourself.

As I wrote in *Losing Your Pounds of Pain: Breaking the Link Between Abuse, Stress, and Overeating,* trying to deny an emotion is like trying to ignore a child who desperately wants your attention. The child screams louder and more urgently until the adult finally acknowledges her. Your emotions are just like that child. If you nurture and pay attention to them, they won't need to scream at you in the form of an overly active appetite. Listen to your food cravings—they are part of your inner voice, and they provide valuable information.

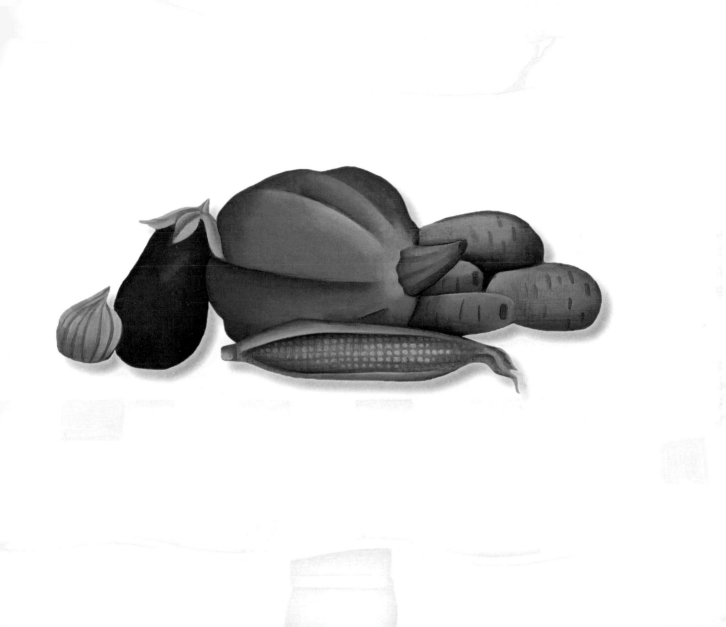

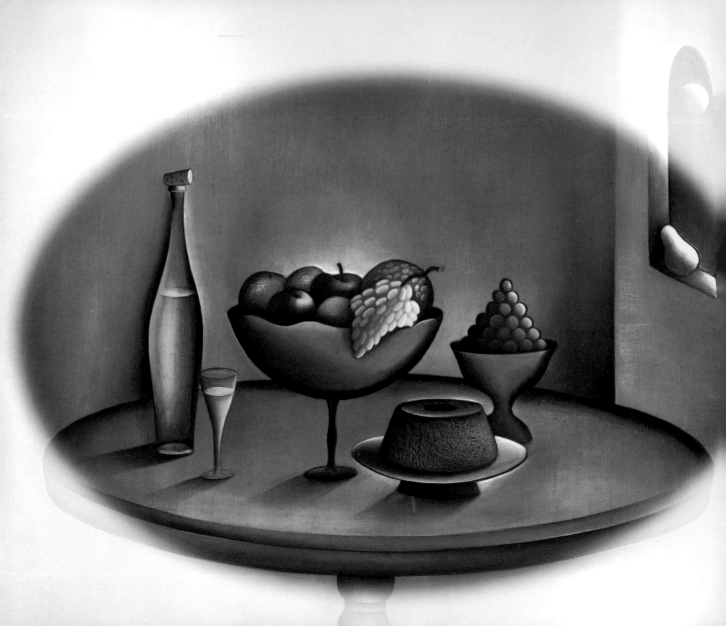

The A–Z Cravings List

What follows is a list of commonly craved foods. It was inspired by Louise Hay's wonderful list of physical and mental challenges found in her books *Heal Your Body* and *You Can Heal Your Life*. This list will help you uncover the underlying feelings triggering your Constant Craving.

I want to remind you that this list refers to food *cravings*, not food preferences. A craving is a persistent and strong desire to eat a particular food. Emotional hunger is intense, sudden hunger that appears in your mind and your mouth. Physical hunger is gradual and occurs in the stomach. This is also different from desiring a piece of cake or a cookie simply because you happen to see or smell that food.

A food craving doesn't originate from contact with the food. Rather, the idea and flavor of the food enters our mind, triggering urges to seek out that food and overeat. They are Constant Cravings, only alleviated by directly addressing the underlying emotional cause.

Each craving is triggered by one or more of the FATS feelings: fear, or its manifestations of anger, tension, and shame. Those are the core feelings that trigger cravings for each particular food.

When we ignore our gut feelings and inner voice, we lose peace of mind. The body attempts to correct this imbalance and return itself to a state of homeostasis, or balanced harmony. If we resist the gut's directions about confronting a troubling circumstance head-on, the body settles for a less satisfactory alternative. Your body knows that if you ingest a certain food, your emotions will be temporarily soothed. Your food cravings urge you to eat the food that matches your emotional circumstance. If you are depressed, you will feel hungry for an antidepressant food. If you are anxious, you will crave a calming food. Your cravings are signals that your body wants you to feel at peace.

Of course, eating food—like taking antidepressant medication—doesn't fix the underlying problem. But sometimes we don't know how to go about modifying our circumstances. We wonder which voice is our inner guide and which voice is just our human desire to control outcomes. All we know is that we feel unsettled and hungry. When you interpret your food craving, you pinpoint which voice belongs to your inner guide.

This A–Z list explains the probable meaning behind your food craving. If the description does not exactly pertain to your current circumstances, try asking yourself, "Am I feeling fear, or its manifestations of anger, tension, or shame right now?" When the true answer comes to you, it will "click." You will know what issue has diminished your peace of mind. Then, ask yourself what action you can take right this moment to begin correcting the troubling situation. Even one small step represents a decision to recover your peace of mind. You will feel better when you make that decision, and your gut will no longer have to seek homeostasis through food cravings.

Affirmations for each food craving are also listed. The stronger and more persistent the craving, the more times you'll want to write and say each affirmation. If you have a negative thought after saying the affirmation, know that this negative thought comes from your fear or its manifestations of anger, tension, or shame. Know that only thoughts born of love are real. Negative thoughts are mental habits that can be healed by consistently affirming these self-loving thoughts for 30 days.

Each time you crave a food, reach for this list and look for the corresponding meaning and healing affirmation. Say the affirmation repeatedly until you feel the craving subside. If you crave a combination of foods, such as those contained in a sandwich, then ask yourself, "Which food within the sandwich am I truly craving?" It could be a combination of five ingredients within the sandwich, so you'll want to look up the meanings for each of those five ingredients. Or, you might realize that only one or two ingredients within the sandwich are what you crave. In this case, you'll only need to read about the single ingredients that you're currently craving. Say all of the affirmations that apply to your current Constant Craving, and you'll soon feel your appetite calm down and subside.

iOi

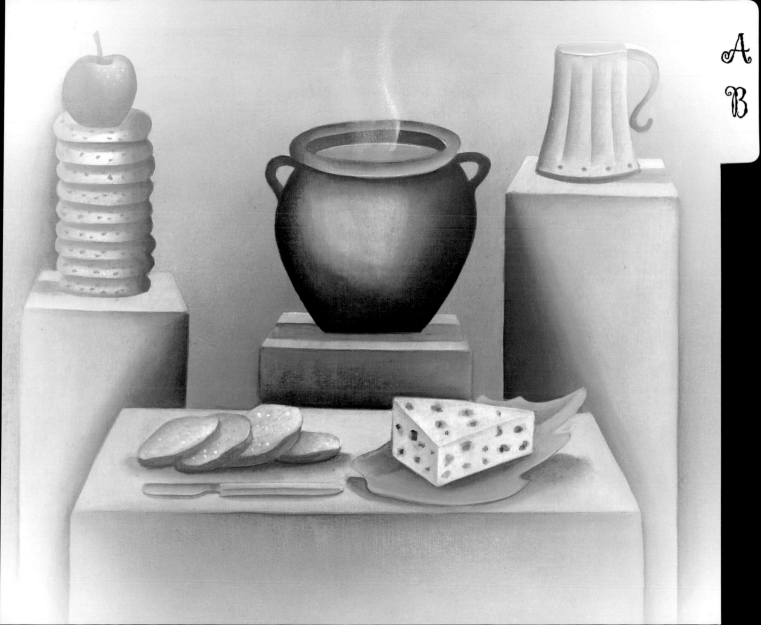

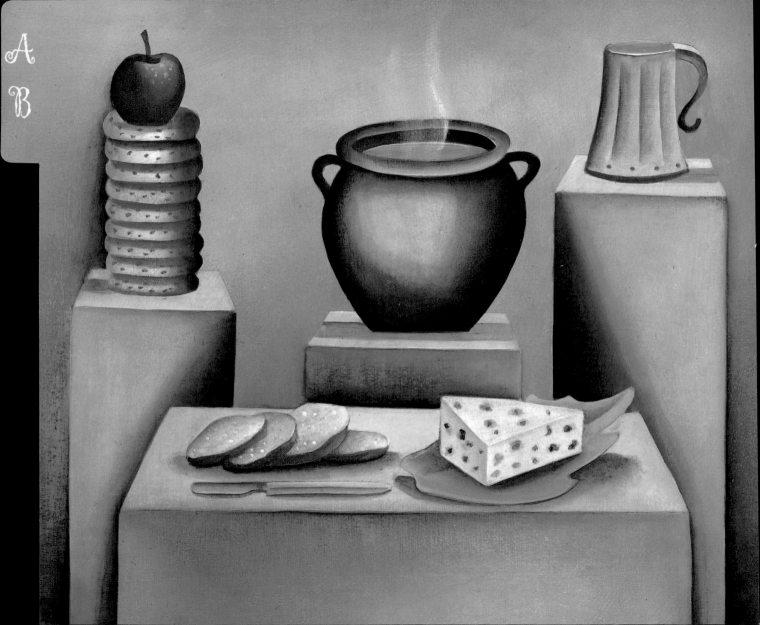

Food Craved	Probable Meaning	Affirmation

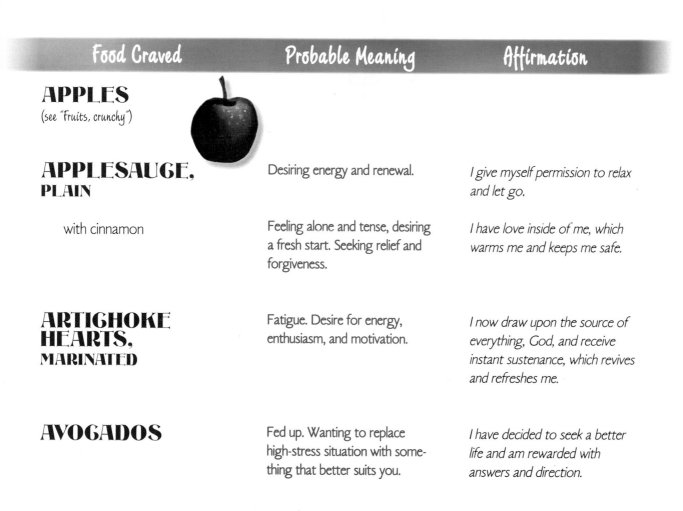

APPLES
(see "Fruits, crunchy")

APPLESAUCE, PLAIN — Desiring energy and renewal. — *I give myself permission to relax and let go.*

with cinnamon — Feeling alone and tense, desiring a fresh start. Seeking relief and forgiveness. — *I have love inside of me, which warms me and keeps me safe.*

ARTICHOKE HEARTS, MARINATED — Fatigue. Desire for energy, enthusiasm, and motivation. — *I now draw upon the source of everything, God, and receive instant sustenance, which revives and refreshes me.*

AVOCADOS — Fed up. Wanting to replace high-stress situation with something that better suits you. — *I have decided to seek a better life and am rewarded with answers and direction.*

BAGON
(see "Pork")

BAGELS
(see "Bread")

BANANAS
(see "Fruit")

BARBEQUE SAUGE
(see "Condiments")

BATTER

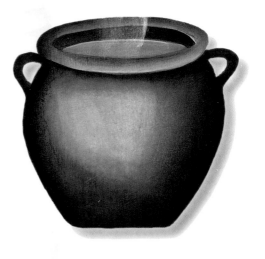

Food Craved	Probable Meaning	Affirmation
cake (chocolate)	Fear of abandonment. Desiring love, hugs, and reassurance.	*God's love is always with me, and I am never alone.*
cake (vanilla)	Insecure and feeling wounded. Feeling afraid and vulnerable to attack.	*Love provides strength and wisdom in all my thoughts and actions.*

Food Craved	Probable Meaning	Affirmation
chocolate chip cookie	Insecure and feeling attacked by love partner. Also, angry at self.	*It is safe to express my true feelings; I forgive and I love.*
pancake	Desiring hugs, but afraid to accept love. Fear of rejection	*I accept the love that is within me; it warms me through and through.*

BEANS, BAKED OR BARBEQUED

	Fatigue. Desire for vacation, time off, change of career, or more fun.	*I now give myself permission to relax and contemplate my inner vision and guidance.*

BEEF

cheeseburger	Frightened of a sense of inner emptiness or inadequacy, and feeling depression. Fear of failure.	*My source of strength source of strength and peace is within me right now. I let go of the belief that I am in control, and put my trust in my Creator.*

29

BEEF (CONTINUED)

Food Craved	Probable Meaning	Affirmation
hamburger	Feeling insecure and unclear. Wanting direction, motivation, and energy.	I release my life to the universe, knowing that God has wonderful plans for me. When I follow these plans, all the details are taken care of.
hot dogs	Desire to return to simpler, more carefree times. Too much responsibility on your shoulders.	I allow my inner child to come out and play. I know that my entire life benefits when I yield to this inner desire for fun.
meatloaf	Desiring comfort, escape, and understanding. Feeling unsafe.	As I radiate love and shine my positive light on my life and others, all negative influences fall away naturally.
pot pie (beef)	Anxiety, worry, and self-blame. Being too hard on self.	I deserve love just for being who I am now.
prime rib	Career burnout. Desire for motivation, energy, and job satisfaction.	I hear and follow my inner guidance, which leads me to right livelihood and greater meaning in my career.

Food Craved	Probable Meaning	Affirmation
• with horseradish	Boredom at work. Desire for a more exciting career.	*I take wonderful care of my emotional and physical self. I balance my schedule and allow time for fun and excitement.*
steak	Tired due to stress. Wanting solutions and energy.	*I have abundant time and energy. The universe has unlimited resources that flow through me now.*
stew (beef)	Feeling attacked and wanting understanding.	*I am gentle and loving with myself. I manifest peace in my mind and my heart.*
stroganoff with beef and noodles or rice	Worry is leading to an energy drain and some self-blame. Wanting relief and energy.	*I have the right to rest and relax. I take time to meet my needs.*

BEER
(see "Liquids")

BERRIES
(see "Fruit")

BEVERAGES
(see "Liquids")

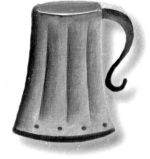

BISCOTTI
(see "Cookies")

BISCUITS
(see "Bread")

BREAD
(INCLUDES BAGELS, BISCUITS, MUFFINS, RICE CAKES, PANCAKES, PASTRIES, AND WAFFLES)

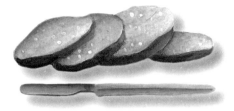

Food Craved	Probable Meaning	Affirmation
toasted plain (crunchy)	Feeling like progress is thwarted. Frustrated.	*I move toward my goals with trust and steady effort.*
• with butter	Feeling trapped; procrastinating making necessary changes.	*I am free to make changes and pursue my Divinely inspired dreams.*
• with banana	Frustrated and depressed. Wanting a miraculous break-through.	*The true source of inspiration is inside of me. I am provided with all the answers I need.*
• with cheese	Anxious about reaching goals and depressed about the future.	*I trust my inner voice and follow its wisdom and direction.*
• with chocolate	Desiring love, support, and encouragement.	*I am strong, loved, and supported.*

BREAD (CONTINUED)

- with cinnamon

Feeling alone or abandoned. Too much to do and not enough help.

I am warmed, knowing that I am enveloped in love. I radiate love outward, and all my needs are abundantly taken care of.

- with cinnamon and raisins

Tension over multiple responsibilities. Fatigue. Indecision about priorities.

My Higher Self is one with the infinite creativity of the Divine mind and the source of unlimited energy right now.

- with garlic (garlic bread)

Desiring escape from an overly intense situation.

I release all my fears and replace them with strength and renewal.

- with honey

Unsure whether you are equipped to take on a task or make necessary changes.

I have the time, talent, and intelligence to accomplish my goals.

- with jam, jelly, or syrup

Tired and overwhelmed. Desiring relief and energy.

I am renewed in mind, body, and spirit. When I follow my inner voice, my enthusiasm is boundless.

Food Craved	Probable Meaning	Affirmation
• with meat, fowl, fish, or lox	Tired and desiring a wave of renewed energy. Frustrated or discouraged.	*I bathe my spirit with the refreshing energy of love and self-approval.*
• with peanut butter, crunchy	Angered by heavy workload; thinking that everyone but you is relaxing and having fun.	*I have the right to ask for help and to take a time-out when I need it. I take care of my need to relax and have fun.*
• with peanut butter, smooth	Not having enough fun. Tired of always putting self last.	*I give myself permission to relax and let go, right now. I deserve to have fun.*
• with pesto	Frustrated by the lack of excitement and fun in your life.	*I am excited by the process of fulfilling my Divine purpose. I am filled with love.*
untoasted (soft)	Insecure and desiring comfort and reassurance.	*I am safe and secure. Love is in me and is surrounding me.*

35

BREAD (CONTINUED)

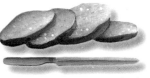

- with banana

  Feeling alone, afraid, and depressed.

  I love myself and know I am never alone when my heart is filled with love. I allow myself to feel good.

- with butter

  Frightened of making necessary changes or taking action. Procrastinating and waiting until you feel more prepared.

  I trust in the Divine Creator who is sowing His plans through me. I know that He will support me completely as I carry out His will.

- with cheese

  Fear and shame. Don't like present situation and afraid to move forward. Fear of failure.

  I am always a success when I allow my inner voice to direct me. I trust that I am Divinely guided.

- with chocolate

  Wanting a love relationship to comfort you.

  Love is reflected in me and around me. I now attract loving people into my life.

- with cinnamon

  Fear and shame. Feeling cold and alone; wanting comfort and love.

  My inner warmth radiates and attracts. My Divine source of love never leaves me. I take action to fulfill my peace of mind.

Food Craved	Probable Meaning	Affirmation
• with cinnamon and raisins	Desiring comfort and security. Homesick. Also, upset due to indecision.	*Within the center of my being, I am always home. My safety and comfort come from following my inner guidance.*
• with garlic (garlic bread)	Feeling bored and left out. Resentment as a result of feeling excluded.	*I am reassured by the knowledge that I am Divinely guided. I am right where I need to be.*
• with honey	Insecure. Fear of rejection, embarrassment, or abandonment.	*I am safe, secure, and loved.*
• with jam, jelly, or syrup	Anger. Hurt feelings. Exhaustion. Desire for comfort and energy.	*I tap into my unlimited source of energy and self-love.*
• with meat, fowl, fish, or lox	Drained, and desiring recharged batteries and emotional support.	*I take excellent care of myself in all ways.*

BREAD (CONTINUED)

- with peanut butter, crunchy

A belief that there is a lack of time. Upset over being pushed too hard, with no fun.

All my priorities are in order. I take a deep breath and gently restore my peace of mind. I look for, and see, humor in my situation.

- with peanut butter, smooth

Depressed and upset that others are having fun without you. Self-pity.

I give myself permission to relax and play. Other people respond lovingly to my requests for help.

- with pesto

Feeling bored and fed up.

I create excitement in my life in healthy, loving ways.

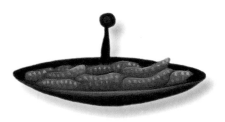

BROWNIES

Desire for romance, yet fearful of a close, intimate relationship.

I am willing to release my fear of giving and receiving love. I trust my inner guide to attract only people who will love, honor, and treat me with complete respect.

BUBBLE GUM
(see "Candy")

BURRITO
(see "Mexican food")

BUTTER
(see "Condiments")

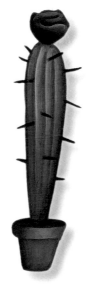

Food Craved	Probable Meaning	Affirmation
BUTTERMILK (also see "Milk")	Desiring energy and reassurance. Distress at having to face a difficult situation.	I center myself in the place within me filled with strength and harmony. I go to that place whenever I face a trying circumstance.
biscuits (see "Bread")		
pancakes (see "Bread")		
ranch salad dressing	Tension. Wanting to relax and feel enjoyment. May feel sad or lonely.	I am surrounded by Divine sources of pleasure, comfort, and companionship.

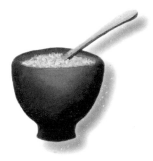

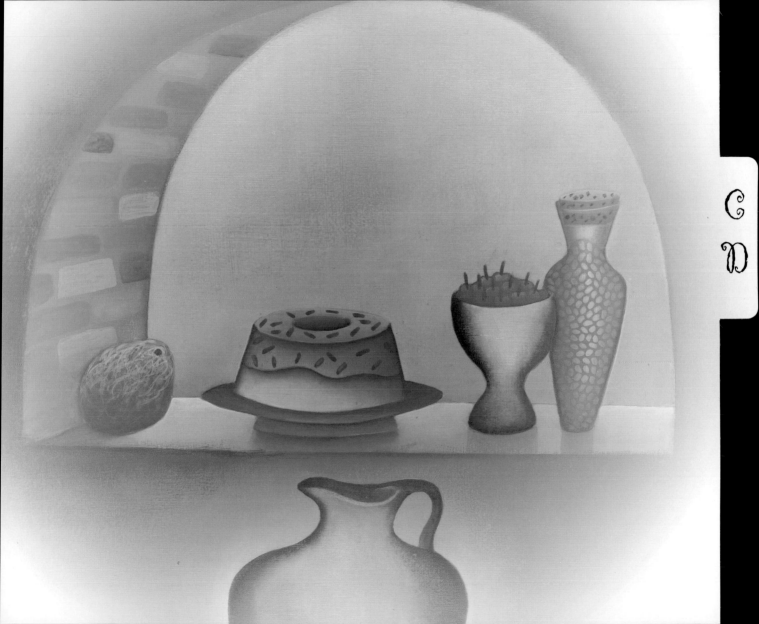

C D

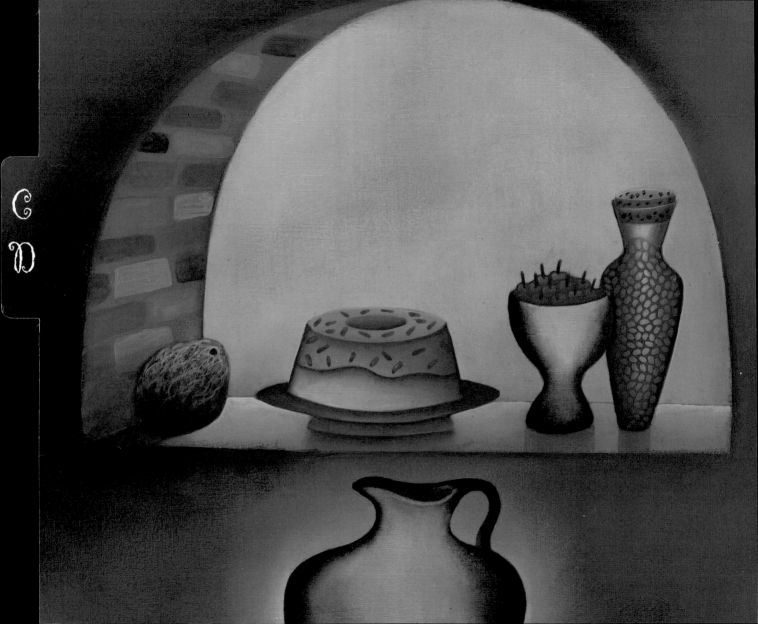

CAKE

angel food or vanilla	Wanting to escape a frightening or stressful situation.	*I know the true source of my power. I relax with the knowledge that my Divine intelligence can be trusted.*
apple-cinnamon	Feeling lonely, withdrawn, with regret, self-blame, and guilt. Wanting forgiveness and relief.	*I feel good about who I am. I know that I deserve love and understanding.*
carrot 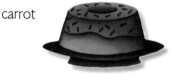	Insecure and worried, either about your job or a family member.	*I face necessary changes with trust, strength, and intelligence. I treat myself gently.*
chocolate	Feeling insecure, possibly due to relationship problems.	*I trust that when I act with love, I am Divinely guided. I am humble and sincere in all my interactions with others.*
chocolate chip	Upset about problems in a relationship. Unsettled by a misunderstanding and harsh words.	*I am soothed by the knowledge that I am never alone. I remain open to love, and I am Divinely directed about my love life.*

CAKE (CONTINUED)

Food Craved	Probable Meaning	Affirmation
chocolate fudge	Desiring escape, and a harmonious union with a loved one. Strong desire for love and comfort.	I reap what I sow, and I am now sowing love in my life. I see the truth in everyone I meet, and know that we are all God's manifestations of love.
chocolate (with nuts)	Wanting more free time, vacations, or nights on the town. Frustrated by lack of love and fun.	I have made a decision to enjoy my life. As I am learning to let go and trust God's plans, I am rewarded with joy and love.
coconut 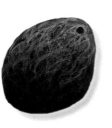	Anxious due to heavy workload, with no end in sight.	I practice self-love when I set a humane schedule for myself. I allow myself breaks and rest time.
coffee cake	Fear. Feeling alone. Desire for warmth, friendship, love, and understanding.	I am enveloped in the warm embrace of reassuring love. My Divine source completely understands and takes care of my needs.

Food Craved	Probable Meaning	Affirmation
German chocolate	Anxious due to a belief that a lack of fun would be cured by the presence of a great love relationship.	I release my need to predict and control. I know that all is well in my life.
pound or shortcake	Wanting to block out awareness of a painful reality. Fear of making a wrong decision.	I have the inner strength to carry on. I act with conviction and make my decisions based on love and wisdom.
tira misu	Desire to shed nerve-wracking tension and replace it with a refreshing wave of energy.	I bathe my soul with cleansing thoughts. My true source of energy begins with my peace of mind.

CANDY

Food Craved	Probable Meaning	Affirmation
Almond Joy	Anger. Bored and angry, or anxious about not having enough fun in love life.	I have the right to relax and have fun. I enjoy this moment now.

CANDY (CONTINUED)

Food Craved	Probable Meaning	Affirmation
bubble gum	Wrestling with indecision. Feeling restless, stuck, excited, and anxious.	I now center my thoughts and emotions in that quiet center within me, where I draw upon the unlimited strength and intelligence that is the truth of my being.
Butterfingers	A desire for friendship and fun, but afraid of rejection.	My friends are loving, fun people who accept me for who I am right now.
caramel	Anxious and drained from excess nervous energy.	I give myself permission to take some time out and listen to my inner voice.
chocolate (in general)	A desire to be filled with the feeling of love.	I am deeply loved right now, and I center myself in this awareness. I am filled with the love of God, and I radiate this love to everyone, everywhere.
chocolate chips	Angry that one's love life is unsatisfactory. Blaming self or others.	My inner source of love is expressing itself perfectly right this very minute; I listen and trust.

chocolate-covered

- cherries

  A desire to relax in a comfortable love relationship.

  All my fears melt as I fall in love with my Divinely guided life.

- coconut

  A desire for love and fun. Envy or jealousy.

  My Divine source of pleasure is inside of me. I give and receive love with pleasure.

- liqueur

  Wanting to block out fears about love life. Desiring comfort and companionship.

  As I receive Divine guidance about my life, it is easy for me to release fears and control.

- nuts

  Frustrated because your love life is boring or nonexistent. Losing patience.

  I have the right to plan my life and take charge of fulfilling my needs.

- peanut butter

  A desire to have more fun in your love life. Wanting nights out, vacations, or dates.

  I follow my heart and find the childlike spirit within me that is the true source of love.

CANDY (CONTINUED)

Food Craved	Probable Meaning	Affirmation
• raisins	Upset that some part of your love life is unsettled or unacceptable.	*I see clearly what needs to be done. I am open to honest discussion and clear communication.*
English toffee	Tension. A desire for complete comfort and frustration about continuous struggles.	*I let go of the need to defend. I am safe and exist without apology.*
fudge, chocolate	An intense craving for love, and feeling an extreme desire for a good relationship.	*I am centered and I radiate love. My peace of mind attracts loving people into my life.*
• fudge (with nuts)	Wrestling with questions about your love life. You're unhappy and resent the way you're being treated, but you worry, "Is it okay for me to feel this way?"	*All my experiences and feelings are valid. I have the right to express my emotions to myself and others. I deserve fun and love.*
Good 'n' Plenty	You feel drained because something worries you. Fear of loss.	*I take action where warranted, and channel worry into free-flowing meditation. Everything has a purpose.*

Food Craved	Probable Meaning	Affirmation
gumdrops	A gnawing worry that haunts you. You want to feel good.	*I know, deep down, that my true beliefs will guide me. I am responsible for listening to my inner voice.*
hard candy (sweet)	Resentment and a block against future prosperity. A desire for revenge.	*I take time to listen to my true voice of reason. I release the need to have any problems, and I revel in the joy of prosperity.*
jellybeans	Worries and insecurity about work; desperately seeking solutions.	*Every one of my needs always has been, and always will be, taken care of.*
• red-hot	Frustrated that you're not experiencing enough excitement or gaining enough recognition.	*I deserve the attention and companionship of others.*
Kit Kat	Your decision not to settle for the wrong mate or inappropriate behavior leaves you feeling lonely or abandoned.	*I approach my love life with intelligence, grace, and love.*

GANDY (CONTINUED)

licorice

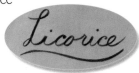

Indecision and confusion. Unsettled due to worry over making the "wrong" choice.

I easily follow my inner guidance, which flows from the source of all intelligence, solutions, and creativity. I trust and follow this guidance now.

M and M's

Work is interfering with your desire to relax and get closer to your mate.

When I let go, all my relationships improve.

• peanut

Your love life is boring and you're angry.

I have fun and love in my life at this very moment.

mint/peppermint/candy canes

Wanting extra energy, alertness, and vitality.

I am refreshed and revitalized right now. I feel terrific!

peanut brittle

Feeling angry or resentful that life is dull or difficult. Feeling like others are blaming you.

I release all beliefs in any kind of difficulty, and affirm the truth of life's lightness and harmony.

peppermint chocolate

Feeling drained because of a contentious relationship; wanting energy and love.

A great love relationship is energizing and refreshing to me. I am now in love.

Food Craved	Probable Meaning	Affirmation
Reese's peanut butter cups	Fear. Wanting more love and fun in your life. Desire for carefree romance.	Today I get in touch with my inner child and let myself feel free and alive.
Snickers	A desire for your love partner to understand your needs. Longing for carefree love, fun, and romance.	I open my heart and connect with my love partner. I drop all defenses and enjoy our togetherness.
Three Musketeers	Tension. Upset about a relationship and confused about how to resolve the problem.	Divine wisdom speaks through me, and my mind stays centered on love.
truffles	Wanting to escape to a pure state of love and bliss.	I am love, and I am in love now.
• with nuts	A deep longing for a storybook romance; wanting to be swept off one's feet.	Perfect love resides within me now. I am complete and I am loved.

GATSUP

(see "Condiments")

CELERY

(also see "Vegetables, crunchy")

Food Craved	Probable Meaning	Affirmation
with cheddar cheese spread	Tension has drained your energy. Desire for celebration.	*I now draw energy and creative solutions from the Divine source, and I feel revived and refreshed.*
with cream cheese spread or ranch-style dip	Tension and fear about the future.	*I surrender my future and all troubling situations to God, and know that the solution is already worked out in truth. I am calm, safe, and loved.*
with peanut butter	Too much work and not enough fun.	*I now give myself permission to relax, laugh, and play. I am in charge of my time, and I delegate in ways that are beneficial to all. When I relax, everyone benefits.*

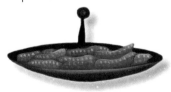

GEREAL

Food Craved	Probable Meaning	Affirmation
sweetened	Dreading upcoming tasks. Desiring energy and a change of circumstance.	I make positive changes when needed. My inner voice always directs me.
• Cap'n Crunch	Resentment over duties or chores. A desire to escape and be free in order to have more fun.	I follow my inner voice's direction toward goals that I naturally enjoy. I balance my life with regularly scheduled free time.
• Cocoa Puffs	Tension. A belief that something is missing, and a desire for more love in one's life.	I relax and allow love to flow through me.
unsweetened/granola	Going through the motions of one's duties with resistance or resentment. Discouraged or depressed.	My purpose is Divinely guided. I listen to, and follow, my inner voice. I embrace changes that bring me closer to God.

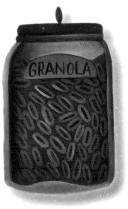

CHEESE

(also see the food that the cheese is served on—e.g., "Pizza," "Nachos," etc.)

mild — Feeling dejected, down, or depressed. Desiring comfort and reassurance. — *I now draw upon the love and energy that comes to me continuously and unconditionally from God.*

sharp — Braced for the worst, and feeling exhausted and drained. A desire for comfort and renewal. Thoughts centered on fear or worst-case scenarios. Weariness. — *My source of energy shines brightly within me. I replace thoughts of fear with feelings of love.*

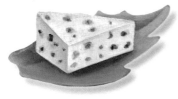

CHEESECAKE

chocolate — Fears concerning a love relationship. A desire to be loved and appreciated. — *I am comforted by my inner source of love.*

Food Craved	Probable Meaning	Affirmation
plain	Fears are triggering some feelings of depression. Wanting reassurance.	*I focus on trusting the Divine wisdom within me. I know that I am guided, and I listen.*
with fruit 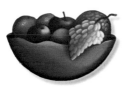	Wanting reassurance and a fresh start. A desire to wipe the slate clean.	*Today I begin a new day and spend each moment in purpose and love.*
with nuts	A desire for friendship and fun. Wanting closeness with others.	*I am a good friend to myself and others. My friends are loving people.*

CHEESE LOG, ROLLED IN NUTS

Wanting stimulation and fun. Reluctance or guilt about having fun.

I embrace today and welcome each opportunity to connect with others.

CHICKEN (AND ALL OTHER POULTRY)

Ala King — Tension. Wanting comfort and energy; feeling drained or depressed.

I am renewed and ready to fulfill my inner vision. I know the right thing to do.

CHICKEN (CONTINUED)

Food Craved	Probable Meaning	Affirmation
baked, broiled, or roasted	A desire for parental love, harmony in the family, and simplicity.	My Divine parent warms my heart and my life with guidance, love, and complete support.
barbequed, crispy	Wanting relaxation and a time-out.	I have the right to relax and enjoy myself.
buffalo wings (spicy)	A desire to let go of concerns and have an exciting, fun time.	Everything in my life is perfect right now. I turn over all my cares and worries to God.
cacciatore or parmigiana	Some frustration is creating an energy drain or depression.	I let go of trying to force a solution. I know that all the answers I seek are within me. When I relax and trust, all my questions are answered.
fried (crispy)	Feeling that goals are thwarted; tired of encountering many roadblocks.	I take a quiet moment to assess my goals. I ask myself, "What is my gut feeling about this situation?"

Food Craved	Probable Meaning	Affirmation
fried (moist)	Self-blame and fear of repercussions. Feeling alone and defenseless.	I am filled with faith and love. I ask for guidance in correcting my thinking about this situation. I forgive myself and let it go.
pot pie (chicken)	Wanting to block out thoughts of problems. Desiring escape and comfort.	I give myself permission to put my worries on the shelf for the evening. I know just what to do.
soup with noodles or rice	Wanting to be soothed and comforted. Feeling hurt or misunderstood.	I focus on the gentle glow of love in my heart and ask it to radiate through me with healing warmth. My burdens are lifted.
with dumplings	Wanting validation, solace, and reassurance.	When I follow my gut feelings and act in accordance, I am rewarded with peace of mind.
with rice (American style)	Tension. Desire to feel lighthearted and carefree.	A breath of spring blows through me, whisking away my cares. I am refreshed and renewed.

CHICKEN (CONTINUED)

with Rice (Mexican style)

Desire for relief from pressure. Life feels complicated and devoid of pleasure.

I release the need to plan and control the outcome. I stay focused on serving God.

CHILI

Desiring excitement and an outlet for stress.

I release my old ideas about how my life is supposed to look. My life is now changing in exciting ways, and I embrace this source of joy.

chili with cheese and/or sour cream

Anger and tension. Stress has built up to the point where you can't see any light at the end of the tunnel. This makes you feel down or depressed, and you long for fun, excitement, and change.

What a relief it is to relax and let go! As I clear away the fog of fear, I am given a clear vision of what I need to do. My life is filled with meaning and joy.

CHINESE FOOD

Food Craved	Probable Meaning	Affirmation
almond chicken	Upset that life is all work and worries and no fun or play.	I have the right to have fun and to play. I give myself permission to schedule recreation into my life.
crispy noodles	Worrying that a situation may backfire or result in a loss.	I am always safe and provided for.
egg rolls	Desire to escape from all worries and stress.	I am comforted by my internal sanctuary, that place inside me filled with omnipotent wisdom and peace.
kung pao (beef, shrimp, chicken)	Wanting more out of life, yet unsure of answers. Frustrated by too much work and not enough rewards.	I take the time now to silently meditate. I ask my inner guide for answers, and I listen with an open heart.
noodles (soft)	Wanting comfort and reassurance.	I fill my entire being with loving thoughts.

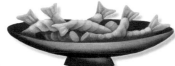

CHINESE FOOD
(CONTINUED)

noodles (spicy)

Wanting more control. Trying to relax after a high-stress day.

I take deep breaths; I breathe out any cares or fears and breathe in delicious feelings of renewal and relaxation.

sweet and sour
(chicken, beef, shrimp)

Fatigue from trying to do too many different things at once. Confusion. Desire for energy.

My life reflects order and peace.

CHIPS
(POTATO OR CORN)

You feel stressed or anxious, and you want to ease your worries. Also, a desire for validation.

I am willing to trust that everything works out for the best. I let go of feeling responsible for everything and everyone around me.

spicy

Overwhelmed, with too many boring responsibilities.

I am open to receiving the lesson in this situation. I follow my joy.

with dip or cheese

Anger and tension. Anxiety or anger that has turned into depression. Feeling betrayed.

I now realize that I am Divinely directed. When I focus on love and joy, I am automatically led away from any source of pain or hurt.

Food Craved	Probable Meaning	Affirmation
with salsa	Tension. You are in a monotonous situation and long for more meaningful or exciting work. Frustration.	I deserve to realize my dreams, which will ultimately make the world a better place. I am ready for changes now.

CHOCOLATE
(see appropriate food category: "Brownies," "Candy," "Ice cream," "Cake," "Coffee," "Doughnut," and "Milk")

COCONUT
(also see "Candy," "Cake," "Cookies," "Pie," and "Yogurt")

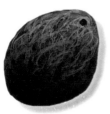

Desire for fun, fulfillment, or rewards for hard work.

It is right for me to follow my inner guidance. It is right for me to take a time out and have fun. When I am relaxed and happy, I positively affect everyone who comes into contact with me.

COFFEE
(see "Liquids")

COLA
(see "Liquids")

CONDIMENTS

barbeque sauce

Boredom. Desire for celebration and break from routines.

I celebrate my life by making each moment and day special. I deserve happiness and rewards.

butter

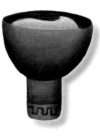

Procrastination. Dreading the start of the day's activities.

I listen to and honor my natural reactions, and I easily adopt changes that allow me to express my desires and natural talents.

Food Craved	Probable Meaning	Affirmation
catsup	Feeling stuck. Searching for answers.	The source of all guidance and directions is within me now. I ask for assistance, and I carefully pay attention to the answers that follow. It is safe for me to take charge of my life.
cornstarch	Fatigue. Desire for increased energy and motivation.	I affirm that my source of energy is now within me, and I choose to become energized by this source right at this moment. I see and feel the energy flowing through and around me, and I feel great right now.
mayonnaise	Desire for comfort and a boost in mood.	I allow myself to honestly face my feelings, and then I release them to God and the angels. I am surrounded by love and assistance, and I willingly accept this help now.

CONDIMENTS
(CONTINUED)

mustard	Feeling deprived. Life feels intense and stressful.	I now choose to allow rewards to come into my life, knowing that I deserve them.
olives	Fatigue. Overwhelming responsibilities.	I ask for help, and others are happy to assist me. I now give myself permission to relax and take a well-deserved rest.
onions, raw; and peppers, hot	Grief and emotional pain. Desire to mask emotions from oneself.	I allow myself to fully express the depth of my feelings, knowing that my healing comes from self-honesty.
pickles		
• dill	Fatigue. Desire for boost of energy.	My source of energy is within me now. I see and feel myself drawing this energy up and around me, and I feel myself instantly revived and refreshed.

- sweet

Sentimental. Concerned about a relationship.

I completely surrender all of my relationships to God and the angels, and I know that they are taking care of everyone's needs right at this moment.

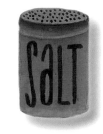

salt

Fear and insecurity. Feeling that you, your position, or your possessions are vulnerable to loss.

I have everything that I need, and it is secure now.

sour cream

Feeling fatigued and blue. Desiring a fresh start and a refreshed outlook.

I now draw upon the energy and enthusiasm that continually resides in the center of my being. I draw upon these resources, and I am refreshed now.

COOKIES

almond, Chinese

Wanting to escape through a fun, yet comfortable activity.

I give myself permission to have fun in all my activities.

COOKIES (CONTINUED)

Food Craved	Probable Meaning	Affirmation
animal	Tension. A desire for more play-time. Feeling a need for rewards and appreciation.	*I delight in my innocence and encourage the child within me to express joy through play.*
batter, uncooked	Feeling vulnerable to attack from others. Also, angry at self.	*It is safe to express my true feelings; I forgive and I love.*
biscotti	Job-related tension.	*I allow my inner sense of timing and direction to lead me in all situations. I breathe deeply and I am refreshed.*
butter	Procrastination. A desire for peace of mind and comfort.	*All my cares are melting away, and my heart is now filled with love.*
chocolate	Tension and fear. Braced for relationship problems. Aching for love.	*I release this problem to you, dear Lord. You know what I need better than I do.*
chocolate chip, crunchy	Tension and anger. Irritated at love partner.	*I open my heart to forgiveness so that love can heal our relationship.*

Food Craved	Probable Meaning	Affirmation
chocolate chip, soft	Frightened that love relationship may be irreparably damaged. Fear of change or rejection.	I let go and trust that my life is changing for the better.
chocolate chip, with nuts	Tension and fear. Upset that love relationship is unfulfilling.	I now seek avenues to increase the love in my life. I attract wonderful, loving people.
cinnamon	Feeling cold and lonely. Frightened of the future.	When I surrender my life to God, only good can happen.
fortune	Braced for problems.	I expect only the best, and that's what I receive.
gingerbread	A desire for simplicity.	My life is clear and full of joy.
lemon	Tension. A desire for friendship.	My friends are loving people who reflect my values and beliefs.
macaroons (coconut)	Wanting time out for play and rewards for hard work.	I allow myself to meet my needs for fun and recognition. I ask for what I want, and I receive it willingly and gratefully.

67

COOKIES (CONTINUED)

oatmeal	Wanting direction in making a decision.	*The source of my answers is within me. All I have to do is ask and then listen.*
Oreos	Tension and shame. Punishing self for perceived lack of love.	*I have decided to put my life back on course, and am reward-ed with abundance and love.*
peanut butter, crunchy	Tension. Frustrated by a lack of fun.	*I am redesigning my life, and it is beautiful and filled with joy.*
peanut butter, soft	Feeling guilty for relaxing, yet feeling sad because life isn't fun.	*Fun is my Divine right. I now ful-fill my need for joy and renewal.*
shortbread (see "Butter cookies")		
sugar	Tension and fear. Wanting to hide from stress and problems. Procrastinating instead of taking action.	*I am safe and secure.*

Food Craved	Probable Meaning	Affirmation
CRACKER JACKS	Resentment because others are interfering with your pleasure.	*All my actions reflect my higher self, and I express my needs with love.*
CRACKERS	Tension. Indecision or trying to feel good about a situation that was thrust upon you.	*This is important. I allow myself to breathe deeply and consider my situation.*
with cheese or dip 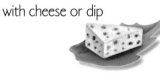	Feeling depressed because an unwanted situation was forced or manipulated onto you.	*I have the right to look at this situation and make my own decisions.*
with peanut butter	Upset because you must work so much when you'd rather be playing and having fun.	*I enjoy this moment right now and know that I am free.*
with salsa	Upset because life seems routine and monotonous. You are craving some big-time excitement!	*I find moments that excite me today; I enjoy the wonderful beauty of day-to-day life.*

CREAM OF WHEAT
(also see "Oatmeal")

A desire for reassurance and support. Wanting comfort.

I am open to receiving love from others. I notice small examples of human kindness.

CROUTONS
(see "Bread")

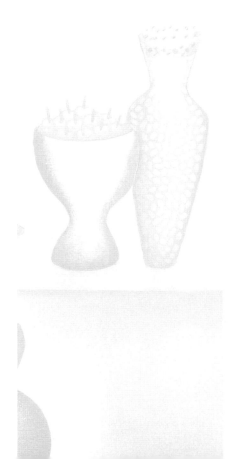

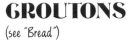

DOUGHNUTS

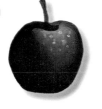

Food Craved	Probable Meaning	Affirmation
apple-cinnamon	A desire for motivation. Feeling dread and trepidation.	*I know the truth about this situation and am willing to make the needed changes.*
chocolate	Anger. Disappointment over love life. Feeling betrayed and desiring comfort.	*My soul is soothed as I prepare to accept love into my life.*
glazed	Drained from being constantly on guard.	*I release my life into the loving arms of my Divine Creator. I ask for, and receive, His protection.*
jelly	Drained by chronic stress and wanting renewed joy and energy.	*I take refuge in my daily silent meditations where I realign my thoughts with what is true.*
with nuts	Desire to replace stress with a carefree life. Resentment or bitterness.	*I release blame and accept good graciously. I give and receive joy.*

DRINKS

(see "Liquids")

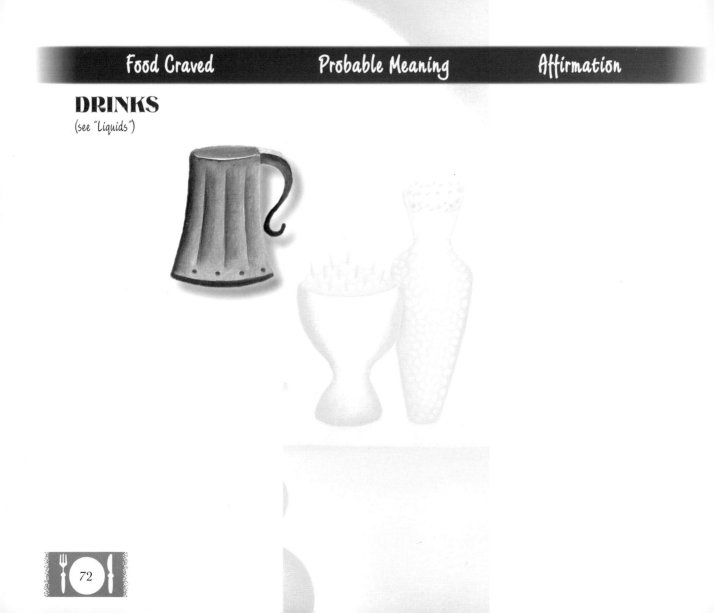

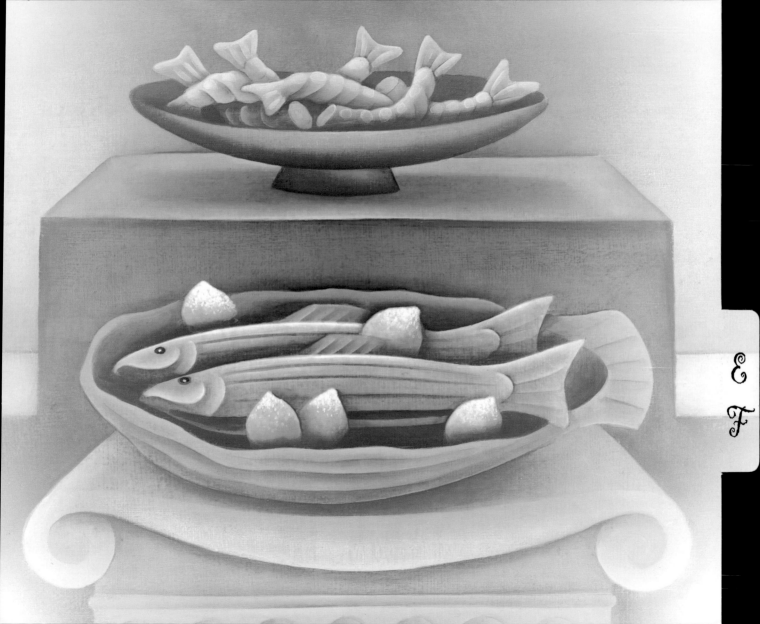

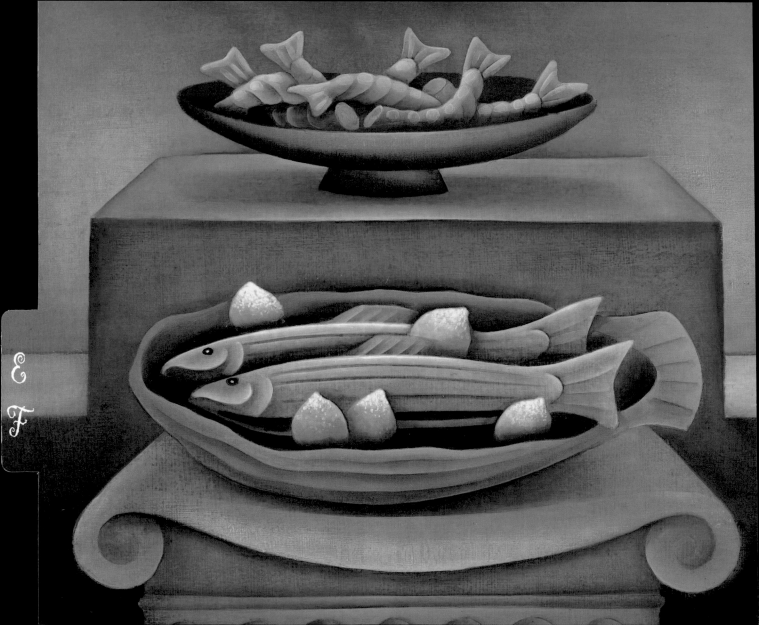

EGGS

boiled	Desire for energy and enthusiasm.	*My source of everything resides within me now. I draw upon this source, and I am revived and refreshed.*
fried/scrambled	Resistance against the day's activities. Dread.	*Whatever I look for, I always find. Today, I look for the fun and love that is hidden within every activity.*
omelette, cheese	Feeling down or depressed about current life situations.	*I have the power to change my life with my thoughts. Today I only think about love, and I receive wonderful opportunities and gifts as a result of these thoughts.*

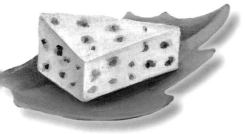

EGGNOG

alcoholic

Burning desire to escape loneliness.

I now see myself surrounded by loving, supportive people. My visualization attracts wonderful relationships into my life.

non-alcoholic

Feeling unloved or misunderstood.

I have wonderful gifts and love to share with others, and I now attract friends and loved ones to me.

ENERGY BARS
(see "Granola bars")

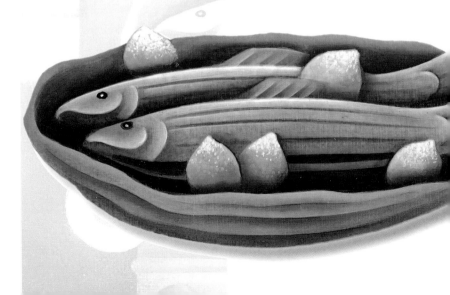

Food Craved	Probable Meaning	Affirmation

FISH/SHELLFISH

baked/broiled	Energy drain from stress.	I take time out to reflect and recharge myself.
deep-fried	Feeling pushed or overworked.	I have decided to make some changes, and that decision provides relief and solutions.
raw	Wanting escape and a new perspective.	I look at my life from all angles, and my creativity is released.
tuna salad	Stressed or worried and wanting to feel secure.	I stay focused on my inner vision and in this way am able to withstand storms.
with butter (melted)	Wanting to feel sure of yourself before beginning an important project. Procrastination stemming from insecurity.	I am filled with the strength of love's direction.

FISH (CONTINUED)

Food Craved	Probable Meaning	Affirmation
with chips, soft; with rice/potatoes/pasta	Energy drain from excessive worrying. Wanting to feel grounded and secure.	*I am comforted when I release my cares to God. He knows the perfect solution to all problems.*
with crunchy chips	Nervousness and concern about an outcome.	*I take a deep breath and say a prayer, knowing that my peace of mind creates positive results.*
spicy/Cajun/Thai	Pressure-cooker or high-risk job drains your energy. Desire to relax and feel certain.	*My enthusiasm is high, and I enjoy learning from my challenges.*
with white sauce	Feeling down or discouraged. Strong desire for comfort and energy; fear of staying discouraged. (This fear perpetuates the discouragement.)	*I deserve the best in all areas of my life. I know that if I can dream it, I can do it.*

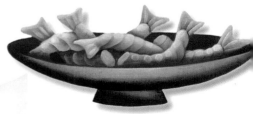

FRENCH FRIES
(see "Potatoes")

FRITTER
(DEEP-FRIED)

A desire for a simpler life; wanting to feel secure and return to one's roots.

I take my time and trust that solutions will present themselves. I slow down and stay open to love.

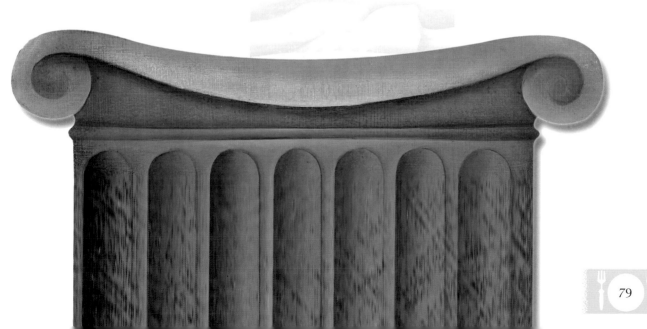

FRUIT

crunchy
(apples, pears, etc.)

Tension. Stress-filled lifestyle is depleting your body's vitamins and minerals.

I nourish my body with love, and schedule time to meet my body's needs.

soft
(melons, peaches, grapes, etc.)

Fear. Overattention to everyone else's needs and not enough toward your own has depleted your body's vitamins and minerals.

I am important and deserve love. When I am healthy and happy, everyone benefits.

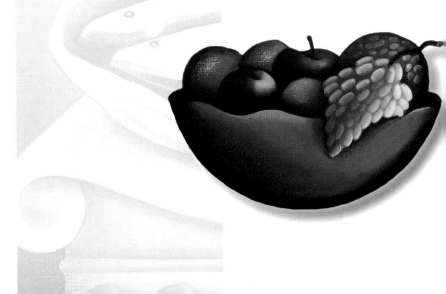

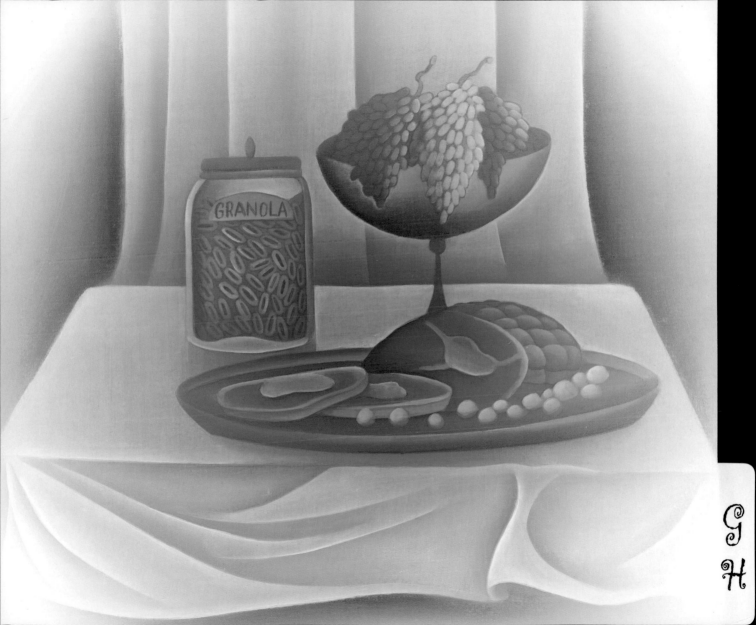

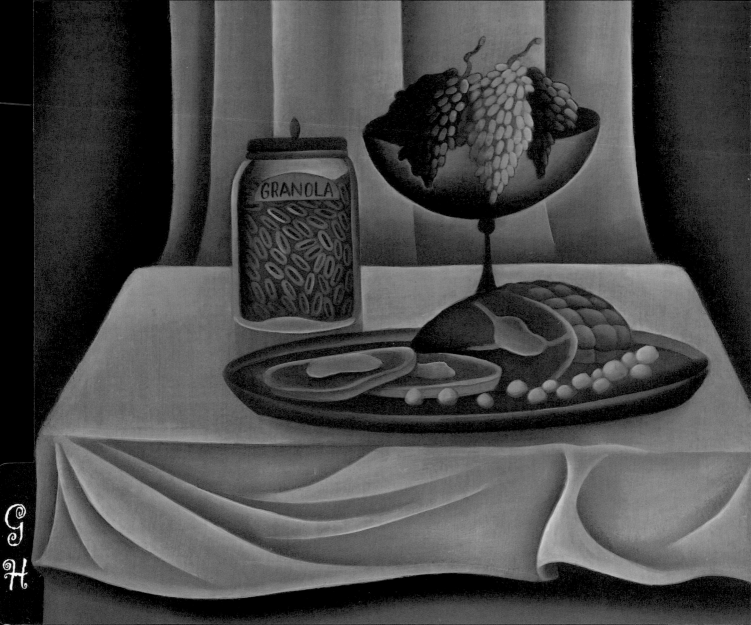

GRANOLA
(see "Cereal")

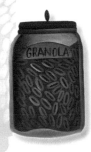

GRANOLA BARS/ ENERGY BARS

Food Craved	Probable Meaning	Affirmation
chocolate-flavored	Frustrated or angered by your love life.	*I now visualize a love life that honors me in all ways, and this vision manifests now.*
cinnamon-flavored	Frustrated and drained because you feel that no one is helping or supporting you.	*My source of help and support is always within me, and I call forth this power to manifest now.*
peanut butter-flavored	Too much work and not enough play. Also, time pressures.	*It is safe for me to relax and enjoy myself. I have an abundance of time in which to get everything done.*

HAM

(see "Pork")

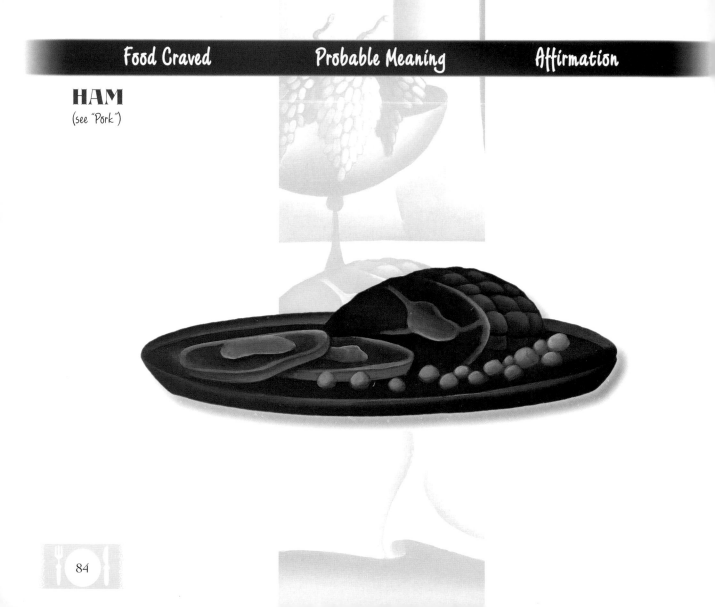

HUMMUS

plain or mild flavor — A desire for energy and enthusiasm. — *I now draw upon the Divine source of all energy, and my soul and body feel nurtured and refreshed.*

spicy — A new project or life change is creating excitement for you. — *I graciously accept change and new blessings in my life. I stay focused in the here-and-now.*

with crackers or other crunchy food — Tension is draining your energy. Also, a feeling of having to compromise your inner desires. — *I am willing to be honest with myself and others, and I trust that Divine love helps me to communicate effectively and with love in my heart.*

with soft tortilla or other soft food — A desire to relax and unwind. A need for a time-out from the day's whirlwind activities. — *I now give myself permission to relax and take a break. I breathe deeply and take my time.*

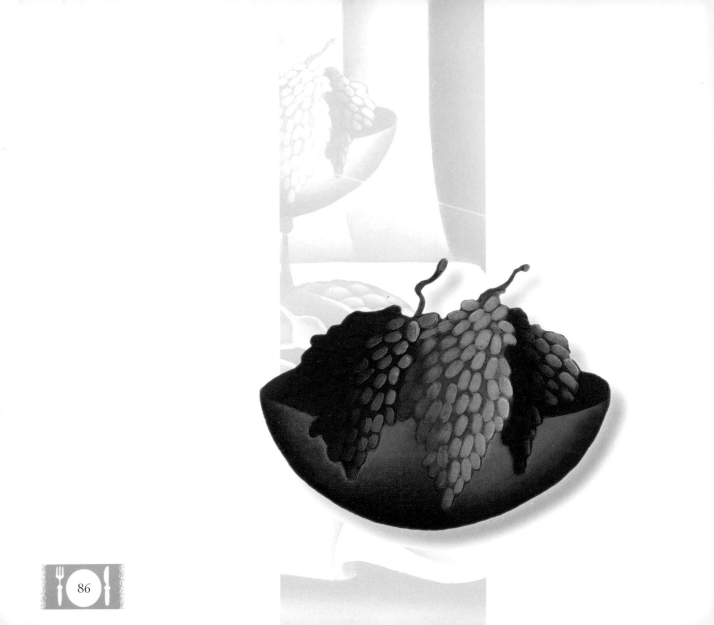

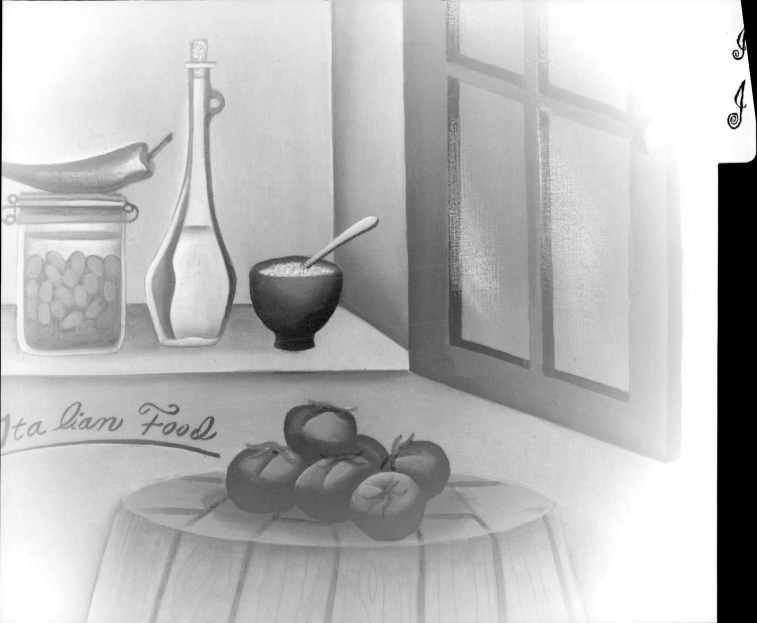

Italian Food

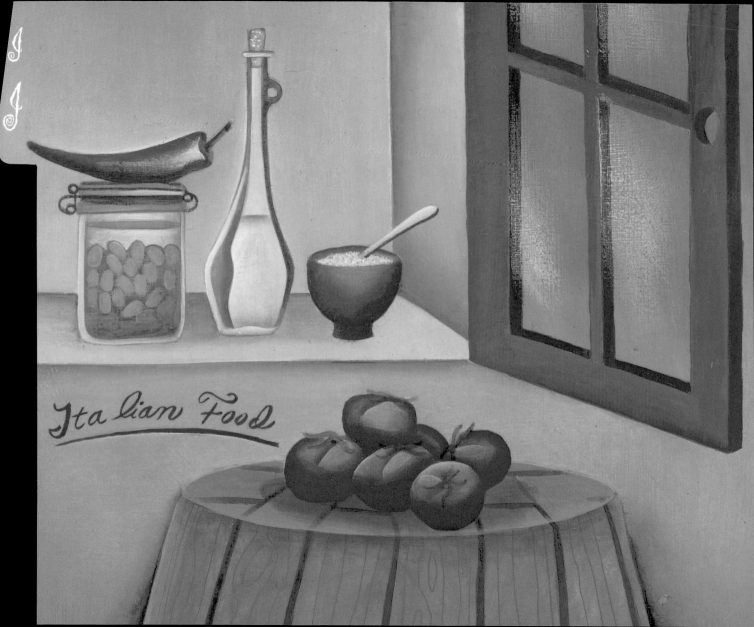

Food Craved	Probable Meaning	Affirmation

ICE CREAM

chocolate	Fear. Disappointment over love life, turned into depression or self-blame.	*Deep down, I have an image of my true love life. I follow my inner guide's direction toward that love.*
chocolate chip	Fear and anger. Feeling angry that love life is unsatisfying, which triggers self-blame and depression.	*I am comforted by knowing that I deserve love. I am open to receiving Divine guidance in all areas of my life.*
coffee	Feeling drained and wanting the incentive to keep going.	*I take a moment to examine my life, and I listen for direction about any needed changes. It is safe to start over.*
double chocolate chip	A feeling that love is being withheld or removed. Frustration that love partner won't change.	*I now let go of fighting and start anew with a soft heart. I bathe my soul in the cleansing comfort of kind thoughts.*

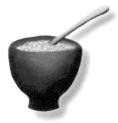

ICE CREAM
(CONTINUED)

Food Craved	Probable Meaning	Affirmation
English toffee/pralines	An upset that has turned into depression or a feeling of being wounded.	*I look for a bright spot of humor in this situation and am surprised by how warmed I am by my own laughter.*
French vanilla	Desire to feel secure and full.	*I am filled with the comfort of God's love.*
Fudgesicle	Feeling wounded by love life; wanting a hug.	*I ask that my needs be met with love in my heart, and my request is always fulfilled.*
mint chocolate chip	Feeling tired and frustrated because of many responsibilities and a perceived lack of love, time, money, or motivation.	*I am renewed by the refreshing love I feel within me right now. I have enough time, energy, money, and motivation to accomplish all my goals.*
mint/peppermint/candy cane	Feeling depressed and drained.	*I allow my inner guide to show me the way to my natural and true state of pure enthusiasm and passion.*

Food Craved	Probable Meaning	Affirmation
peanut butter	Self-pity and disappointment. Lonely for friendships and fun.	*I am a good friend and deserve the love of others. My friends and I share happy times.*
pistachio	Wanting more fun in your life. Depressed that your responsibilities seem endless.	*I clear a space in my heart for pleasure. My joy begins within me now.*
rocky road	Resentment toward others and self. Feeling used or pressured; desiring fun and comfort. Depression.	*I give and receive forgiveness, and my heart softens with love. This love then ensures that all my needs are met.*
sherbet	A desire to unwind or celebrate.	*I shed all worries and replace them with jubilation.*
strawberry	Wanting a fresh start with renewed enthusiasm.	*Right now my life is opening up to exciting new changes.*
vanilla	Tension and fear. Wanting to be soothed and renewed. Also, a desire for optimism.	*I can decide right this minute to embrace the positive forces I feel inside of me.*

ITALIAN FOOD

Italian Food

breadsticks
(see "Bread")

calamari	Tension and fear. Anxious or worried and afraid to face the source of these feelings.	I face life head-on, feeling secure in the knowledge that my inner voice will guide me and keep me safe.
calzone (see "Pizza")		
cannelloni/manicotti/ravioli	Anger and shame. Feeling powerless to make needed changes. Feeling trapped and depressed in high-stress job.	I now reclaim my power and strength, which is fueled by truth and love.
garlic bread	Feeling bored and left out. Resentment stemming from feeling excluded.	I am reassured by the knowledge that I am Divinely guided. I am right where I need to be.

Food Craved	Probable Meaning	Affirmation
lasagna	Trying to block awareness of emotional pain. A desire to shield oneself from attack.	*My vulnerability is my greatest strength because humility keeps me receptive to God's voice.*
pasta (plain)	Wanting comfort and reassurance.	*I fill my entire being with loving thoughts.*
• with alfredo or extra cheese	Discouraged and wounded. Desire for empathy. Guilt or self-blame is blocking the receipt of good.	*I graciously accept good into my life, knowing that I deserve pleasure, support, and love.*
• with marinara	Resentment is causing distress.	*I let go of all blame and focus on solutions.*
• with meat or fish	Wanting comfort and renewed energy.	*My true source of energy comes from following my heart and inner guide.*
• with pesto	Wanting escape and excite-ment. Dreaming of time off or a vacation.	*I decide to give myself a break and schedule some free time into my day.*

93

ITALIAN FOOD
(CONTINUED)

- with pine nuts

Feeling time pressures and resentment toward others. Wanting more fun.

Today I look for moments of pleasure, fun, and enjoyment. I give myself the gift of laughter.

pizza (crispy crust)

- with extra cheese

Feeling afraid of the future. Reluctant or insecure.

I give myself permission to trust.

- with extra meat

Feeling desperate for renewed energy or enthusiasm.

I am filled with hope with respect to the fulfillment of my inner vision.

- with spicy toppings/anchovies

Tension, fear, and shame. Insecurity masked by workaholism. Drained from constant adrenaline highs.

I deserve the best in life. I face my dreams head-on, knowing that I deserve them.

- with "the works"

Drained from financial insecurities. Desire for abundance.

I now experience abundance in all areas of my life. God is a loving parent who wants the best for all His children.

94

Food Craved	Probable Meaning	Affirmation
Soft or regular crust		
• with extra cheese	Depressed or discouraged; wanting reassurance.	I am calmed by the eternal presence of love deep inside me. I feel warmed all over.
• with extra meat	Energy drain from fears or insecurity.	I am good, I am safe, and I am loved.
• with spicy toppings/ anchovies	Confused and feeling out of touch with true feelings. Wanting pleasure and relief.	It is safe for me to enjoy myself.
• with "the works"	Struggling with lack in one's life. Feeling ripped off and yet having difficulty believing you deserve better.	I release the need to have lack in my life.

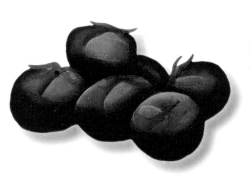

JUICE
(also see "Liquids")

fruit

Desiring energy, rejuvenation, and a time-out from a hectic schedule.

I allow myself to follow my inner sense of timing and direction. I breathe deeply and I relax as I fulfill my purpose in life.

vegetable

Some fear and insecurity about your future is draining you.

I am willing to release all blocks that keep me from enjoying full faith. With faith, I know that all things are possible and that my needs are continuously and abundantly met.

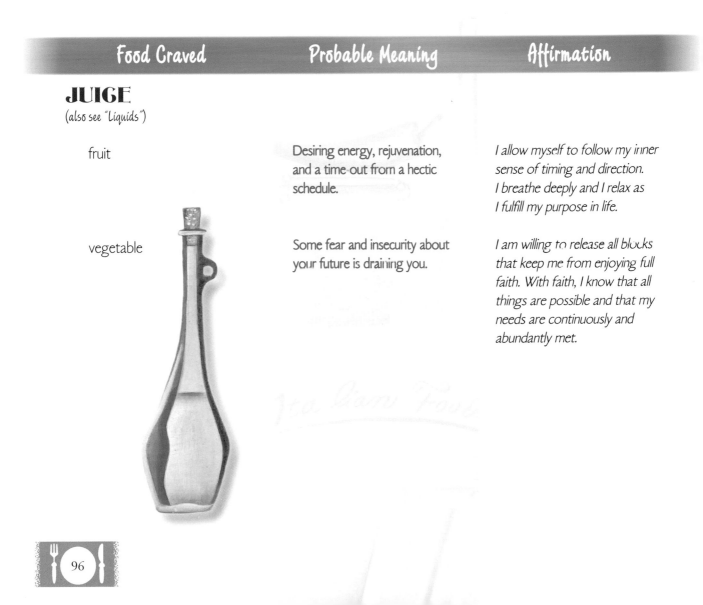

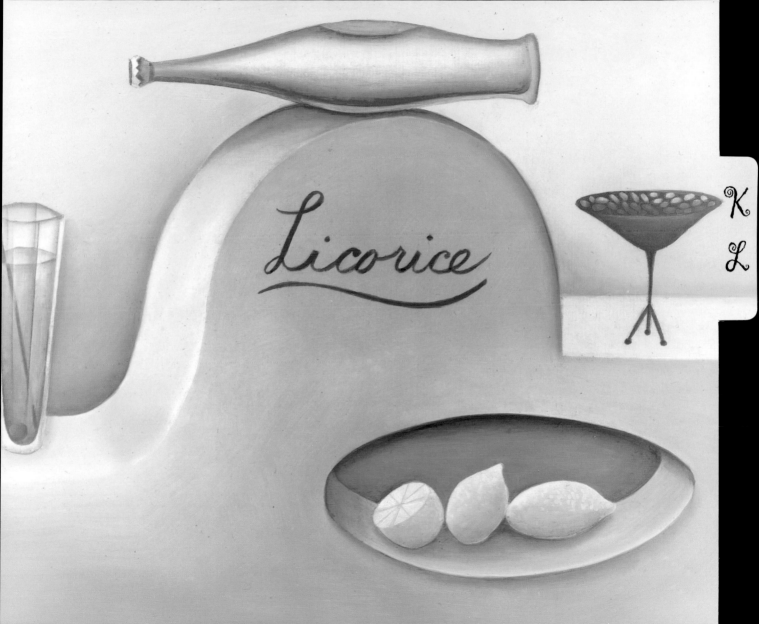

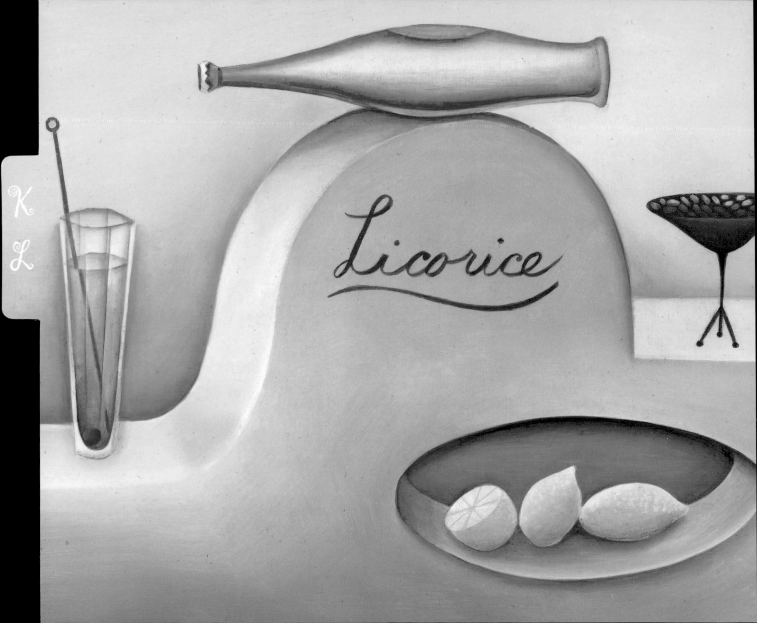

Licorice

Food Craved	Probable Meaning	Affirmation
KABOBS, GRILLED MEAT WITH VEGETABLES	Desire for energy and celebration. Searching for peace and meaning with your career.	I allow my heart to guide me to the place within me where all joy, meaning, and energy exists.
KASHI		
as breakfast cereal with milk	Frustrated or angry about the tasks that are before you.	I now take responsibility for every part of my life, and I choose to live and create a life of pure joy.
as pilaf	Desire for fulfillment. Fear of making a wrong decision.	I listen to, and follow, the steps that my inner guide gives to me. It is safe for me to move forward.
KEY LIME PIE (also see "Pie")	Seeking time-out from chaotic lifestyle.	I deeply breathe in peace, and I am centered in tranquility now.

KUNG PAO
(also see "Chinese Food")

Wanting more out of life, yet unsure of answers. Frustrated by too much work and not enough rewards.

I take the time now to silently meditate. I ask my inner guide for answers, and I listen with an open heart.

KIM-CHI

Fear of the future. Also, grief. Feeling numb. Can also signal alcohol abuse.

I am now willing to surrender my fears to the spiritual help that always surrounds me. I allow my fears to be lifted and replaced with a new feeling of peace and contentment..

LAMB
WITH MINT JELLY

Feeling unappreciated at work. Hard work with low rewards is sapping your energy.

I give myself a pat on the back. I know that I am a valuable person.

LASAGNA
(see "Italian Food")

Food Craved	Probable Meaning	Affirmation
• mint	Wanting to recharge your batteries. Desire to feel refreshed and reenergized.	I visualize a stream of white light through the center of my being, and I draw upon this energy to awaken me completely.
• pekoe, hot	Wanting a time-out to contemplate your thoughts.	I take a deep breath, close my eyes, and give my full attention to my inner guide.
with milk or cream	Feeling pushed by a schedule that exceeds your comfort level.	It is right for me to set my own pace according to my inner guide's direction.
with sugar	Desiring rewards or acknowledgment for hard work.	I now drink in all of the love that resides within me. It feels good to know that I have made a wonderful difference in the lives of many people.
• pekoe, iced	Seeking creative solutions and new ideas.	I now allow the creative expression of my higher self to fully express itself without reservation.

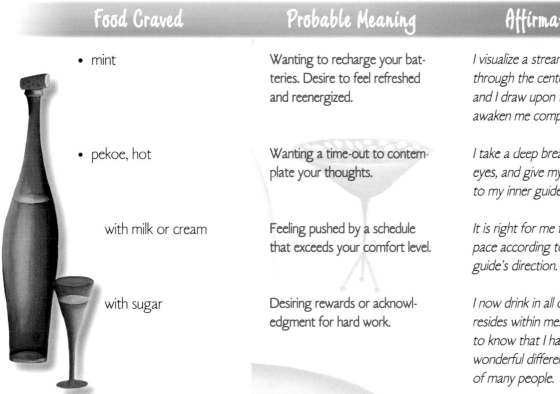

LIQUIDS (CONTINUED)

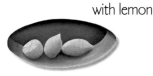

with lemon

Wanting more motivation to face and complete an undesirable task.

I am an unlimited being, and I am free to soar to the greatest of heights.

with sugar

Boredom. Wanting to attend an exciting event or celebration.

I take charge of my emotions, time, and environment. I am willing to release any fears I may have about living an exciting and meaningful life.

LIVER,
BATTERED AND FRIED

Financial and/or familial insecurities are creating feelings of emptiness.

I am filled with the gifts of Spirit, and I draw upon those gifts now. Everything I need is provided for me.

LOBSTER

without butter

Desire for success. Strong aspirations, accompanied by anxiety about current situations.

I am successful and happy now. All of my dreams flow toward me, in partnership with my higher self and God.

Food Craved	Probable Meaning	Affirmation
with drawn butter	Disappointment with income from current job. Procrastination at taking action to resolve financial situation.	I now see myself as successful and motivated. I make meaningful money doing meaningful work.

LOLLIPOP
(also see "Candy")

Food Craved	Probable Meaning	Affirmation
bitten or chewed	Blaming others or the world for your stress or challenges.	I am willing to forgive everyone, including myself, in exchange for everything I want. I am free, and I am filled with happiness and new ideas.
slowly dissolved in mouth or licked	Feeling lonely, bored, or discouraged.	My heart is filled with love, which I now extend to others. I know that I receive what I give, and I now give the gifts which I desire to have, as well.

LONDON BROIL
(also see "Beef")

Dreaming of goals and a "better tomorrow." Future orientation, instead of enjoying the here-and-now.

I capitalize upon the joys and possibilities that are given to me in this very moment.

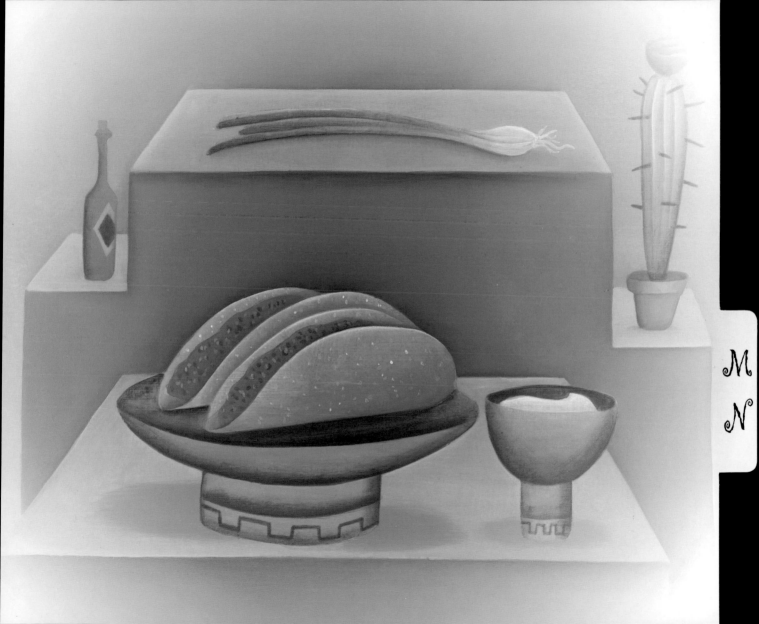

M
N

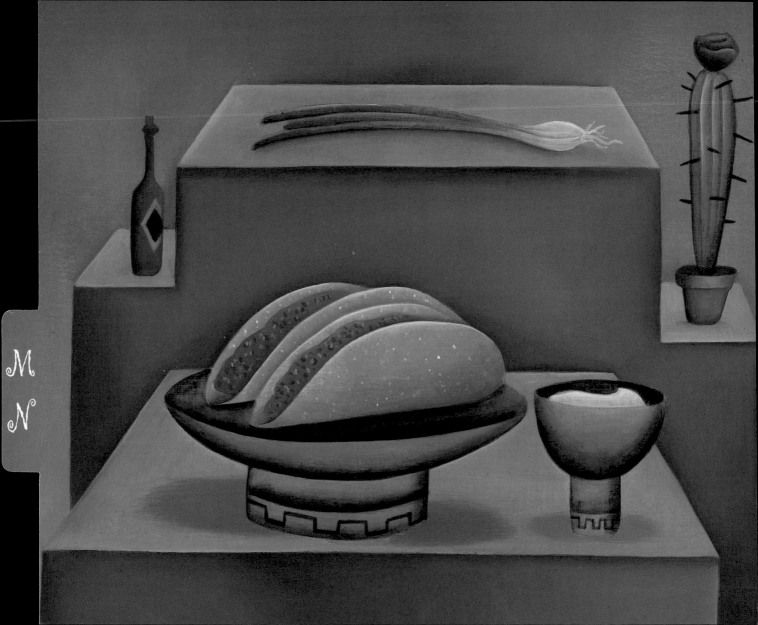

Food Craved	Probable Meaning	Affirmation

MACARONI AND CHEESE

Wanting reassurance and comfort. Feeling attacked, alone, or powerless.

I have the strength of God within me now. I am willing to release all fear of owning my God-given power. I am Divinely guided as I use this power and strength for the good of humanity, including myself.

MAYONNAISE
(see "Condiments")

MELON
(see "Fruit, soft")

MEXICAN FOOD

crunchy (tacos, nachos, tostadas, etc.)

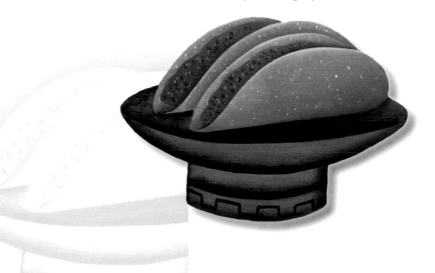

MEXICAN FOOD
(CONTINUED)

Food Craved	Probable Meaning	Affirmation
• with extra cheese or sour cream	High stress in a mismatched job. Depression.	I have the right to make changes in my life. When I follow my inner guide, I am always safe.
• with extra meat	Energy drain from futile struggles or an unworkable situation.	It is such a relief to let go of struggling! When I relax and trust, I am rewarded with peace of mind and abundance.
• with extra salsa	Resentment; feeling trapped. Anger at self.	I have the right to change my life to fulfill my dreams.
soft (burritos, chili rellenos, etc.)		
• with butter	Fear of making a "wrong" decision. Procrastination. Feeling stuck.	I ask for Divine guidance to help me know which choices to make, and I allow myself to act upon this guidance without delay. I surrender my fears to God, and the angels that now surround me.

Food Craved	Probable Meaning	Affirmation
• with extra cheese or sour cream	Feeling like a punching bag for others.	I surround myself with love. I am kind to myself, and others treat me with respect.
• with extra meat	Despondent over feeling victimized.	I am victorious in fulfilling my Divine destiny. My present and future are bright and strong.
• with extra salsa	Self-blame over unhappiness.	I ask for, and receive, respect and assistance.

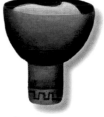

MILK
(see "Liquids")

MINT
(also see "Candy," "Ice Cream," and "Tea")

Desire for some extra energy. Wanting to be wide awake and alert.

I visualize the white light of God's energy within me now, and I ask that this light become stronger and brighter. I now feel revitalized and energized.

Food Craved	Probable Meaning	Affirmation
NUTS (ALL VARIETIES, SALTED OR UNSALTED, ROASTED OR RAW)	Tension. Too much stress and not enough fun=anxiety and lowered peace of mind.	*It's okay for me to relax and play. I give myself permission to have fun.*
barbeque-flavored	Desire for celebration or party with friends or family. Chomping at the bit to have fun and let your hair down.	*I now see myself having a great time with my loved ones, and this vision manifests into form at the perfect time.*
hot and spicy	Vacation is long overdue, and anger about overwork is near the boiling point.	*I now allow myself to take a time-out, knowing that by so doing, I am better able to fulfill my purpose in the world.*
sweet or honey-roasted	Desire for more rewarding responsibilities. No fear of hard work; however, a fear of meaningless work.	*I take charge of my life, and I add meaningful projects to my day's activities. I am inner-self directed, and I trust this guidance now.*

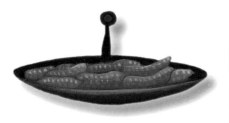

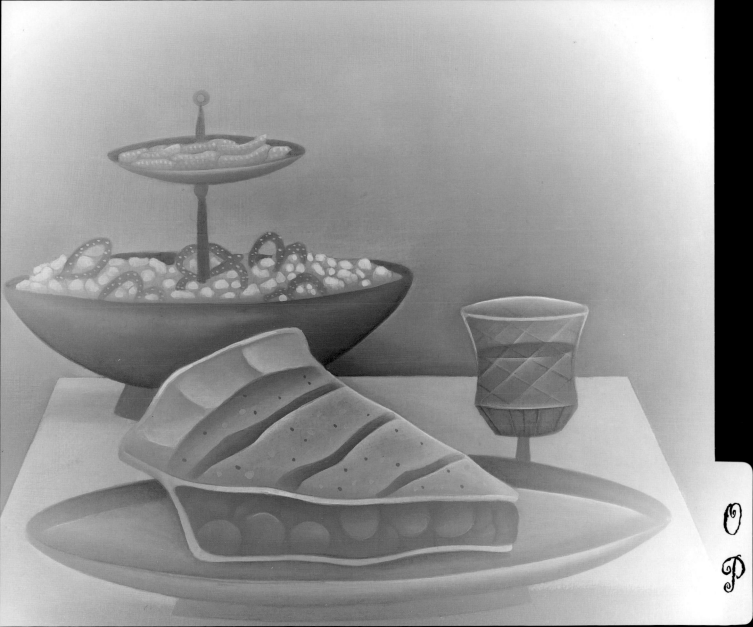

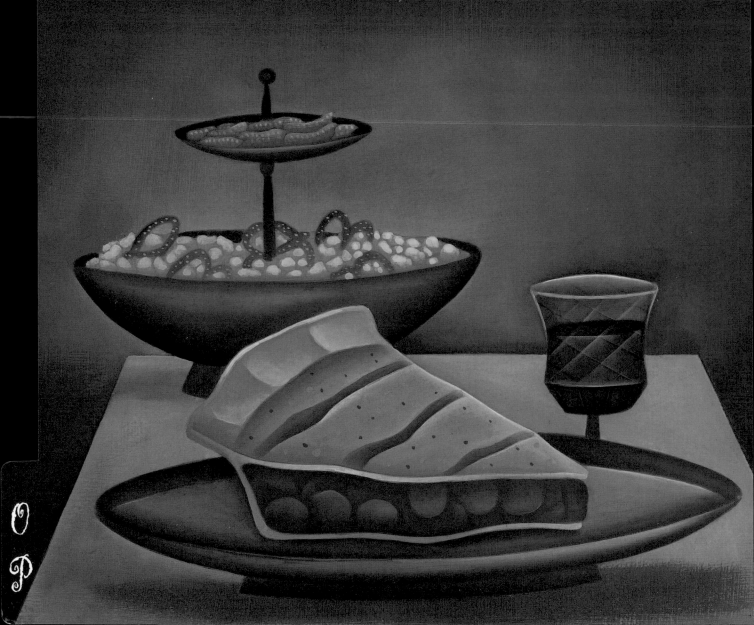

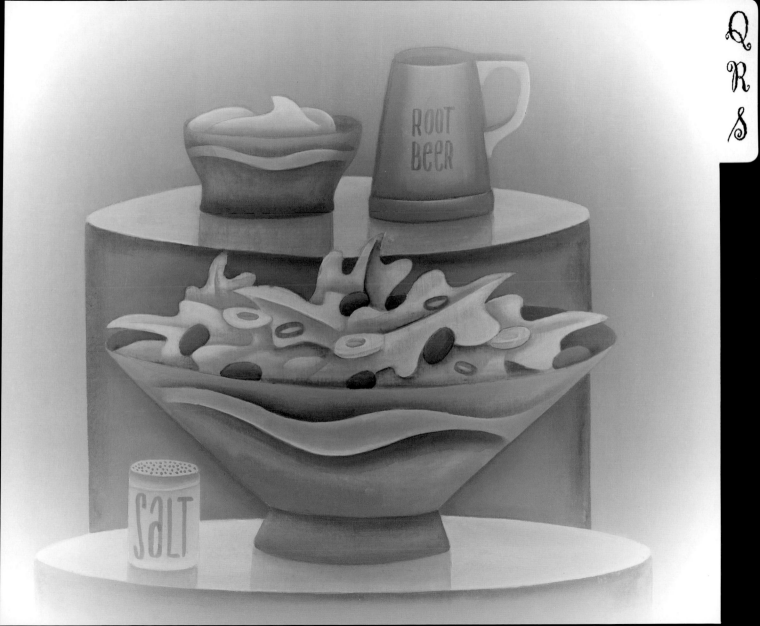

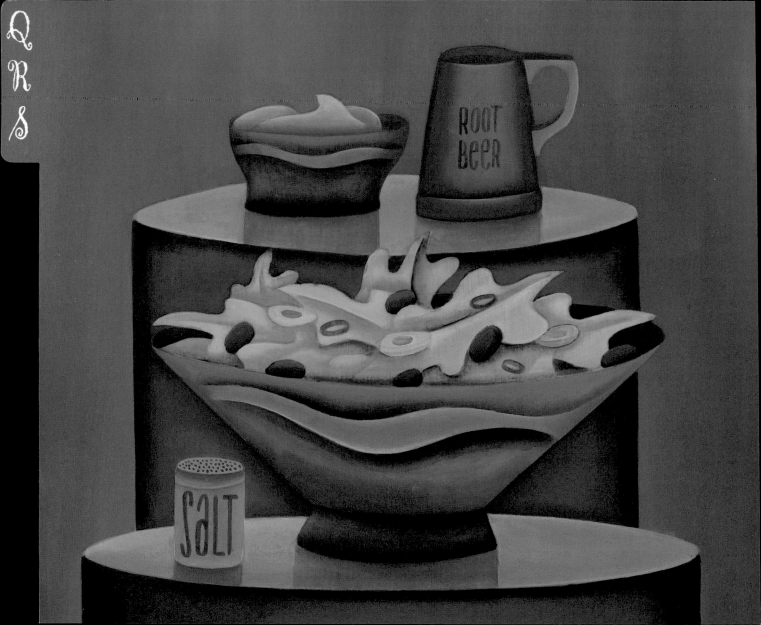

Food Craved	Probable Meaning	Affirmation
RAISINS	Indecision. Wrestling with making a choice.	*I now tune in to the universal intelligence that resides eternally within me. I allow my creativity and Divine direction to guide me now and always. My Divine source cannot err.*
RICE		
brown, whole-grain, wild rice (unseasoned)	Hectic schedule or stress has depleted you, and you have a desire to slow down and rest.	*I have an endless supply of energy, enthusiasm, and time right now.*
pilaf/Rice-a-Roni (seasoned)	The day's activities were too intense for your tastes. Desiring some time to sort things out.	*As I breathe in, I take in the delicious taste of relaxation. As I breathe out, I let go of anything that weighs upon my mind.*
stir-fried, Chinese style with egg	Feeling pushed beyond your comfort zone. Wanting to slow down the speed of changes in your life.	*I have an abundance of time, and I allow myself to move at the pace that my inner guide directs. I trust that others will understand why I must follow my inner clock.*

133

RICE (CONTINUED)

white (steamed or boiled)

Desire for feelings of stability and security.

I am filled with the love of God that resides within me, now and always.

with butter, melted

Procrastination. Wanting to put off working on a dreaded activity.

It is safe for me to admit my feelings to myself. I am willing to speak and act upon my truth.

with soy sauce

Sentimental for the "good old days" or times past, which seem to be better than your present life.

I now allow myself to enjoy every moment, knowing that life is filled with gifts and opportunities.

SALAD

(see "Avocados," "Croutons," "Onions," "Salad dressing," and "Vegetables")

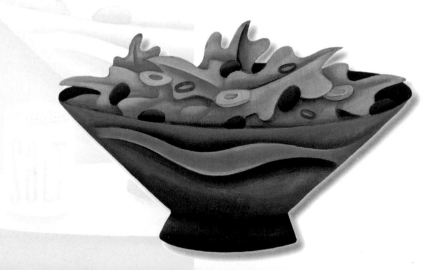

| Food Craved | Probable Meaning | Affirmation |

SALAD DRESSING
(also see "Condiments")

creamy, dairy-based (blue cheese, French, ranch, Roquefort, Thousand Island, etc.)

Desiring true inner happiness. Depression, exasperation, or frustration.

All of my emotions are intelligent and honest. I honor and listen to my feelings.

honey-mustard

High stress level and/or hectic schedule has you desiring some time out.

I listen to my needs, and I ask my inner guide for guidance on meeting these needs.

vinegar-based (balsamics, Italian, vinaigrettes, etc.)

Desire for motivation. Feeling burned out or bored.

My feelings are the starting place that lead me to honestly assess my goals and desires. I face all of my feelings with trust and an open mind.

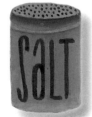

SALT
(see "Condiments")

SEAFOOD
(see "Fish/shellfish")

SMOOTHIES
(see "Liquids")

SODA
(see "Liquids")

SOUR CREAM
(also see the food on which the sour cream is placed—e.g., "Mexican food")

Feeling fatigued and blue. Desiring a fresh start and a new outlook.

I now draw upon the energy and enthusiasm that continually resides in the center of my being. I draw upon these resources and I am refreshed.

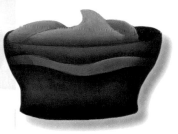

SOUP

broth-based meat, poultry, or seafood

Desire for stability and security.

I am warmed by the sure and certain knowledge that God always provides for and protects me. I am safe.

Food Craved	Probable Meaning	Affirmation
• with rice or noodles	Wanting comfort and reassurance. Feeling disjointed from the world.	*My higher self is filled with love, and I drink in as much love as I desire.*
broth-based vegetable	Stress has left you feeling cold and drained.	*My inner source of eternal love warms and energizes me right now.*
• with rice or noodles	Fear of the future. Desire to avoid facing circumstances head-on.	*I am perfectly guided by God, my higher self, and my angels. I am never alone, and I am always safe.*
cream-based seafood or poultry (e.g., cream of chicken, clam chowder, etc.)	Feeling defeated, especially concerning your work life.	*I visualize success in all of my endeavors, knowing that my thoughts create my reality.*
cream-based vegetable (e.g., cream of broccoli, cream of mushroom, etc.)	Desiring a retreat from a hectic life.	*Deep within me, all is calm, and I am perfectly centered in peace and harmony.*
tomato (non-cream-based)	Ambition is waning; desiring motivation and energy.	*I am willing to release any fears I may have about being a powerful person.*

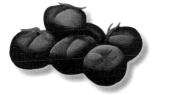

SOUP (CONTINUED)

with crackers (all soup types)

Anxiety, tension, or frustration, in addition to the meaning stated next to soup type.

I now choose to adopt a peaceful outlook, and this blankets me in serenity and centeredness.

SUSHI

Tired of feeling bored.

I follow my joy and create a new life for myself.

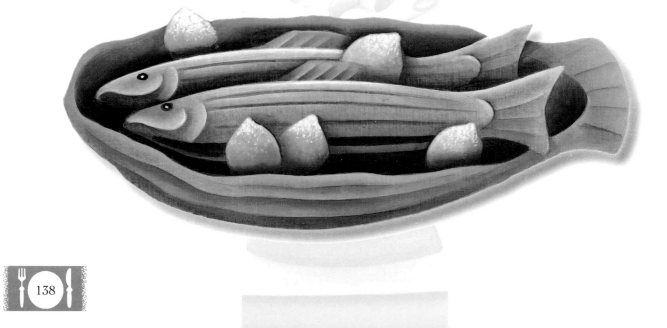

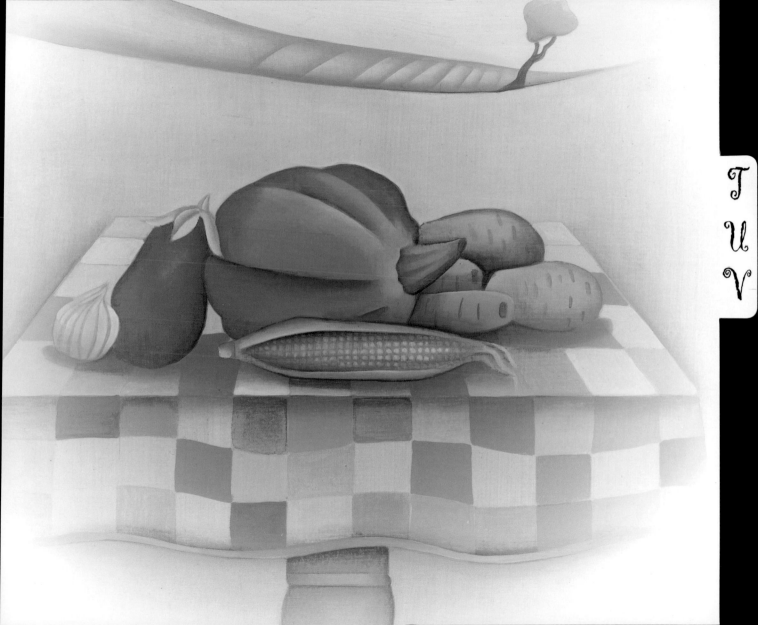

TUV

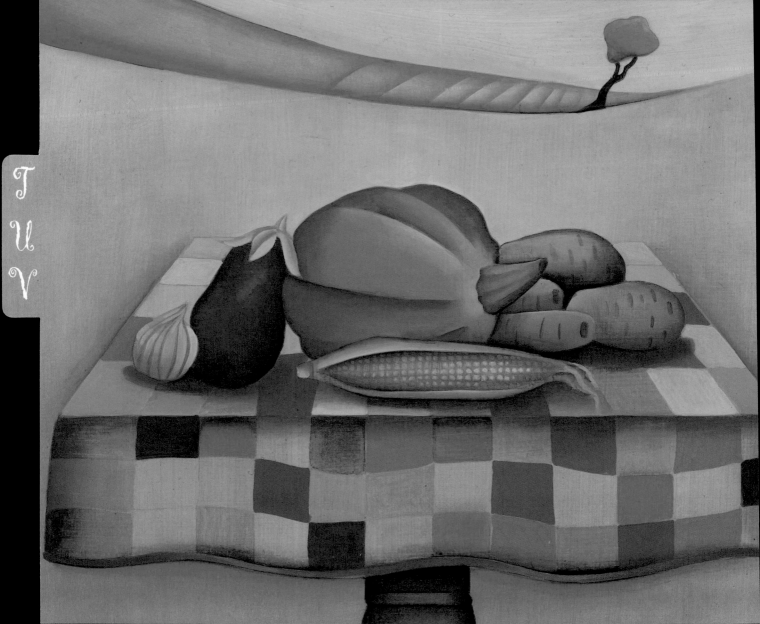

TEA
(see "Liquids")

TOAST
(see "Bread")

TOMATOES
(see "Vegetables")

TOSTADA
(see "Mexican food")

TURKEY
(see "Chicken")

VANILLA
(see appropriate category—
e.g., "Candy," "Ice Cream")

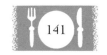

141

VEGETABLES

crunchy
(also see "Celery")

Tension. Stress-filled lifestyle is depleting body's vitamins and minerals.

I nourish my body with love, and schedule time to meet my body's needs.

soft
(also see "Avocado")

Fear. Overattention to everyone else's needs and not enough focus on your own has depleted your body's vitamins and minerals.

I am important and deserve love. When I am healthy and happy, everyone benefits.

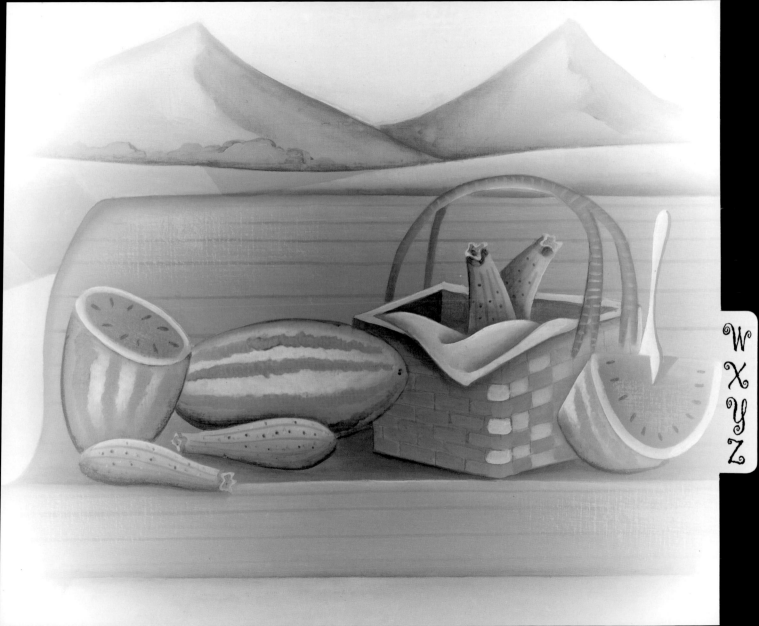

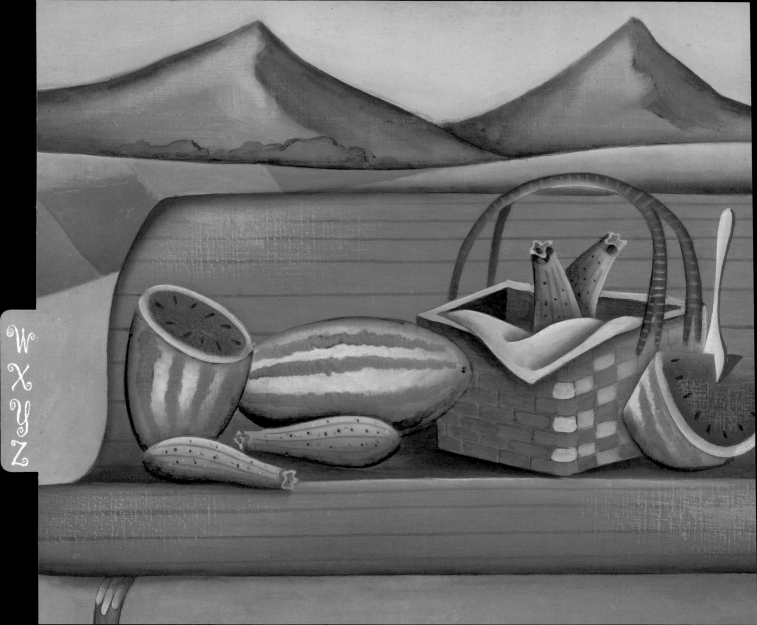

WALNUTS
(see "Nuts")

WATERMELON
(see "Fruit, soft")

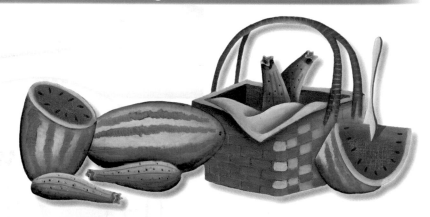

YOGURT
(for toppings, see "Candy," "Granola," "Fruit," or "Nuts")

chocolate-flavored	Feeling disappointed in your love life. Desiring more romance.	*I am willing to release any fears I may have about giving and receiving love.*
chocolate mint-flavored	Wanting an exciting and romantic adventure.	*I now give myself permission to enjoy the love and companionship of others.*

YOGURT (CONTINUED)

Food Craved	Probable Meaning	Affirmation
coconut-flavored 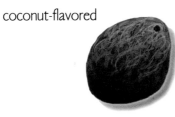	Boredom is making you feel blue.	I ask that God and my higher self use my natural talents and interests in a meaningful way so that I may make a positive difference in the world.
fruit-flavored	Desiring a fresh start and a renewed outlook.	I have everything I need right now. I draw upon my eternal source of energy and enthusiasm, and I am instantly revived and refreshed.
peanut butter-flavored	There's too much work and not enough fun in your life.	I now give myself permission to play. I see my life as balanced and harmonized, and it is so.
vanilla	Resistance to moving forward or making changes. Desire to keep the status quo.	I take the time to meditate upon my alternative futures. I choose a future in which I am engaged in meaningful activities. I feel safe and loved.

ABOUT THE AUTHOR

Doreen Virtue, Ph.D., is a metaphysician who holds B.A., M.A., and Ph.D. degrees in counseling psychology. She gives workshops across the country on intuition, spiritual healing, and manifestation. Doreen has appeared on *Oprah, Good Morning America, Leeza,* CNN, and other shows; and her work has been featured in *McCall's, USA Today, Woman's Day, Redbook,* and other publications. For information on her workshop schedule or to contact Doreen, please call or write the Hay House publicity department, or visit Doreen's website at **www.AngelTherapy.com.**

Also by Doreen Virtue, Ph.D.

Books

Angel Therapy
Chakra Clearing
Constant Craving
Divine Guidance
"I'd Change My Life if I Had More Time"
The Lightworker's Way
Losing Your Pounds of Pain
The Yo-Yo Diet Syndrome

Audiocassettes

Divine Guidance (audio book)
Chakra Clearing
Healing with the Angels
Losing Your Pounds of Pain (audio book)

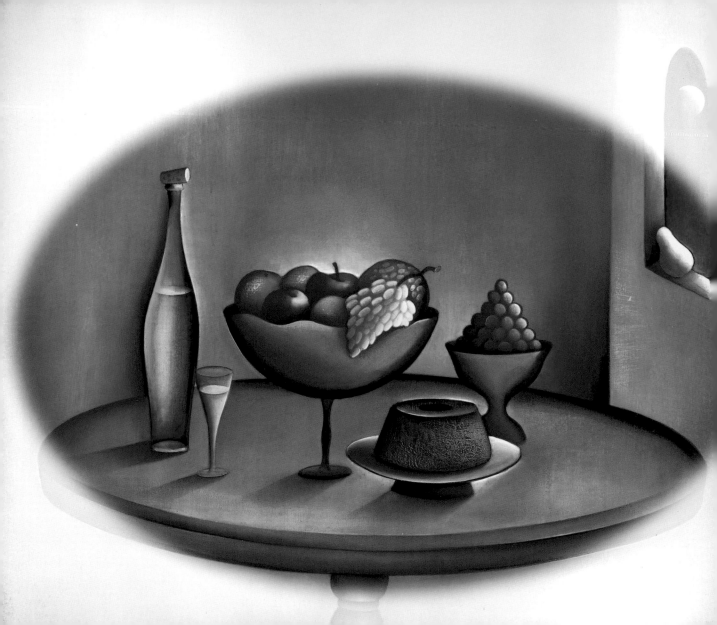

Hay House Lifestyles Titles

<u>Flip books</u>

101 Ways to Happiness, by Louise L. Hay
101 Ways to Health and Healing, by Louise L. Hay
101 Ways to Romance, by Barbara De Angelis, Ph.D.
101 Ways to Transform Your Life, by Dr. Wayne W. Dyer

<u>Books</u>

A Garden of Thoughts, by Louise L. Hay
Aromatherapy A–Z, by Connie Higley, Alan Higley, and Pat Leatham
Constant Craving A–Z, by Doreen Virtue, Ph.D.
Healing with Herbs and Home Remedies A–Z, by Hanna Kroeger
Heal Your Body A–Z, by Louise L. Hay
Home Design with Feng Shui A–Z, by Terah Kathryn Collins
Homeopathy A–Z, by Dana Ullman
and
Power Thoughts Affirmation Cards, by Louise L. Hay

All of the above titles may be ordered by calling Hay House at 800-654-5126

Please visit the Hay House Website at: www.hayhouse.com

We hope you enjoyed this Hay House Lifestyles book.
If you would like to receive a free catalog
featuring additional Hay House books
and products, or if you would like information
about the Hay Foundation, please contact:

Hay House, Inc.
P.O. Box 5100
Carlsbad, CA 92018-5100

(760) 431-7695 or (800) 654-5126
(760) 431-6948 (fax) or (800) 650-5115 (fax)

Please visit the Hay House Website at:
www.hayhouse.com